Pulses & Grains

Your Guide to

Healthy Eastern Mediterranean Style Recipes

A Vegan Cookbook

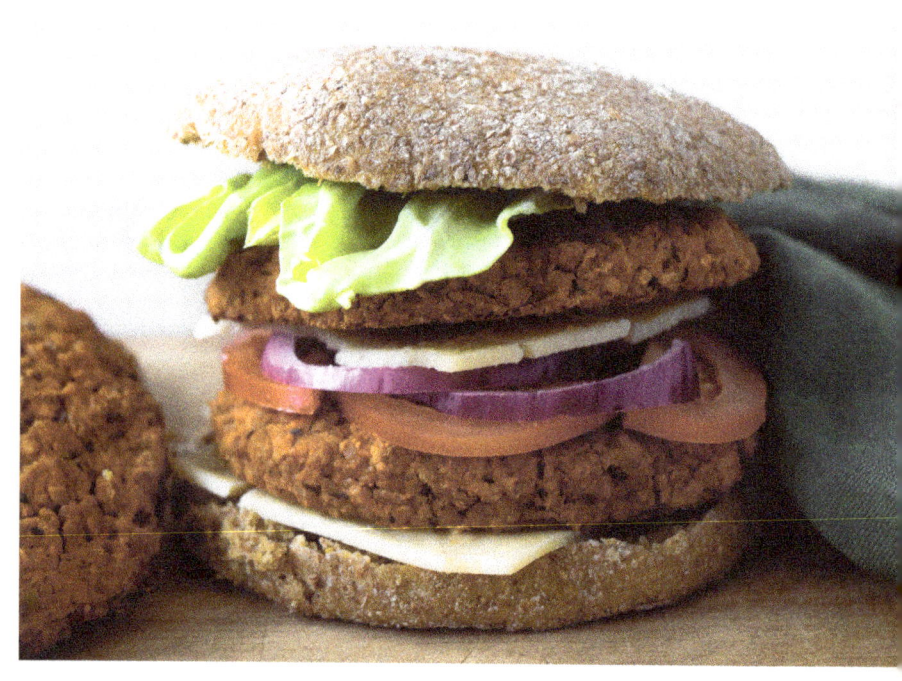

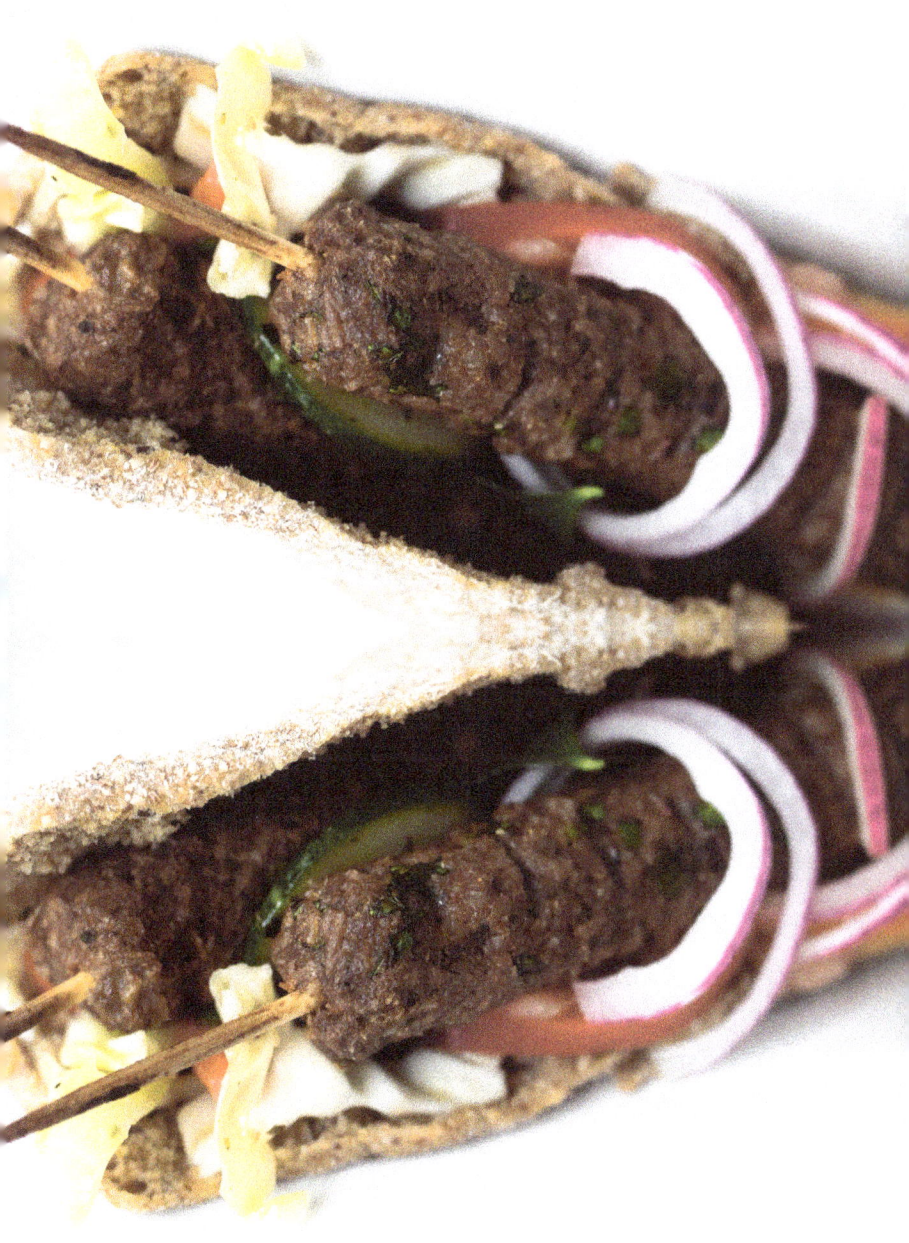

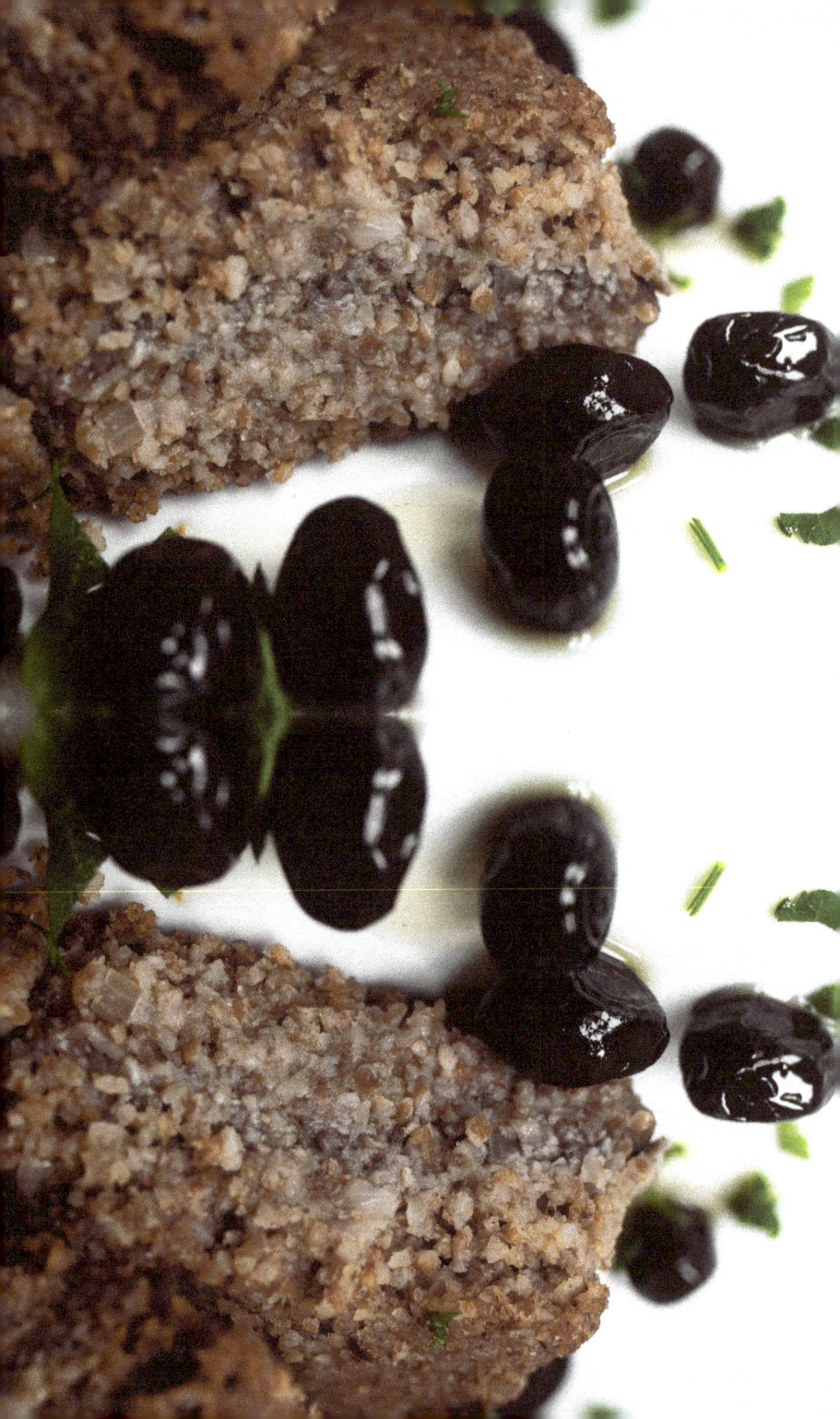

These recipes…

- are affordable and accessible for all individuals and families
- include functional herbs such as thyme, sage, mint, parsley and dill
- are energy saving (by cooking a large number of pulses, then storing or freezing for later use)
- provide options to use minimal spices or no spices at all, for people who do not like spice or are sensitive to them
- are rich with Mediterranean flavours, herbs, spices and nutrients
- are cooked to preserve nutrients and are free of hydrogenated and animal fat
- have been developed and designed on the East Mediterranean/Levant region cuisine

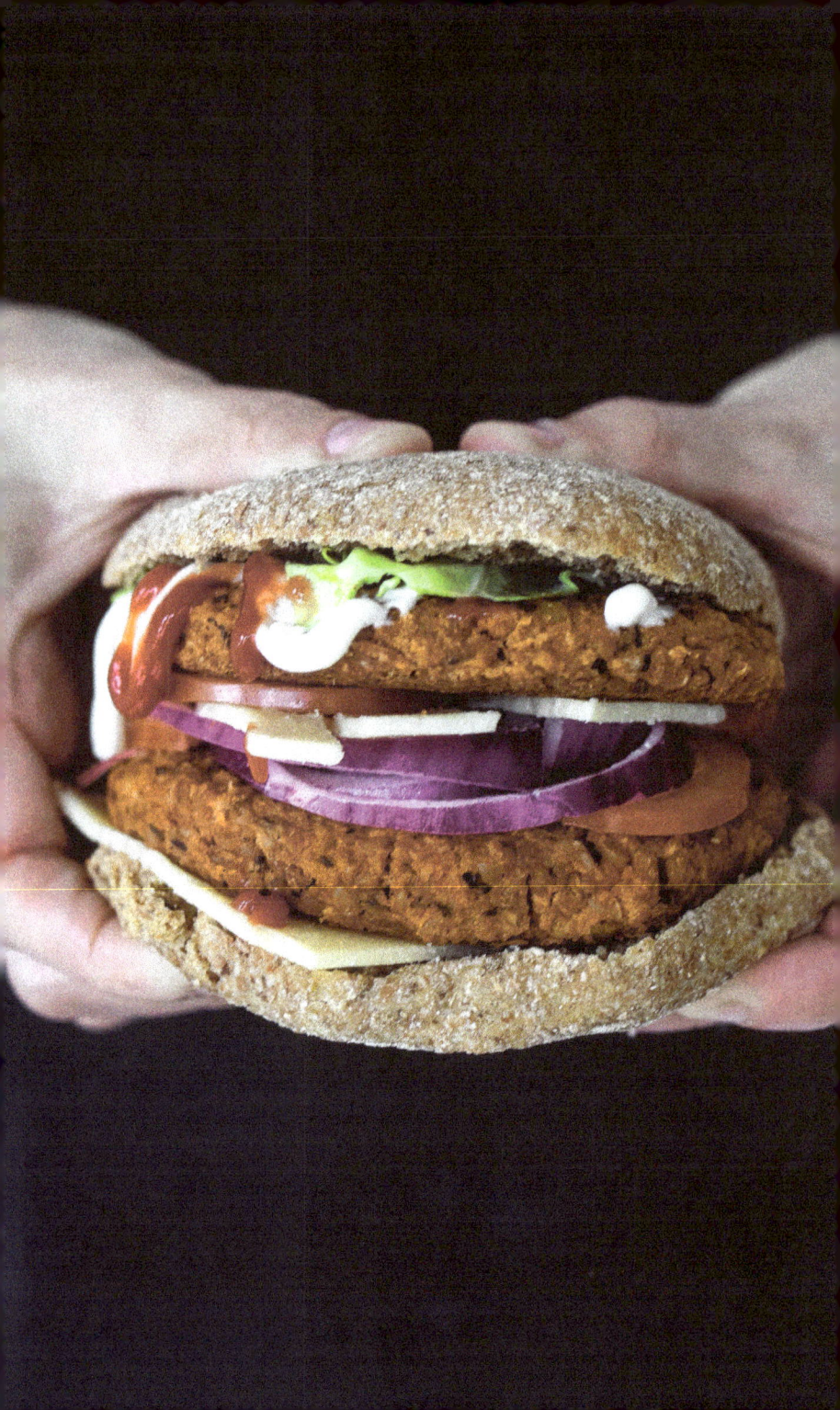

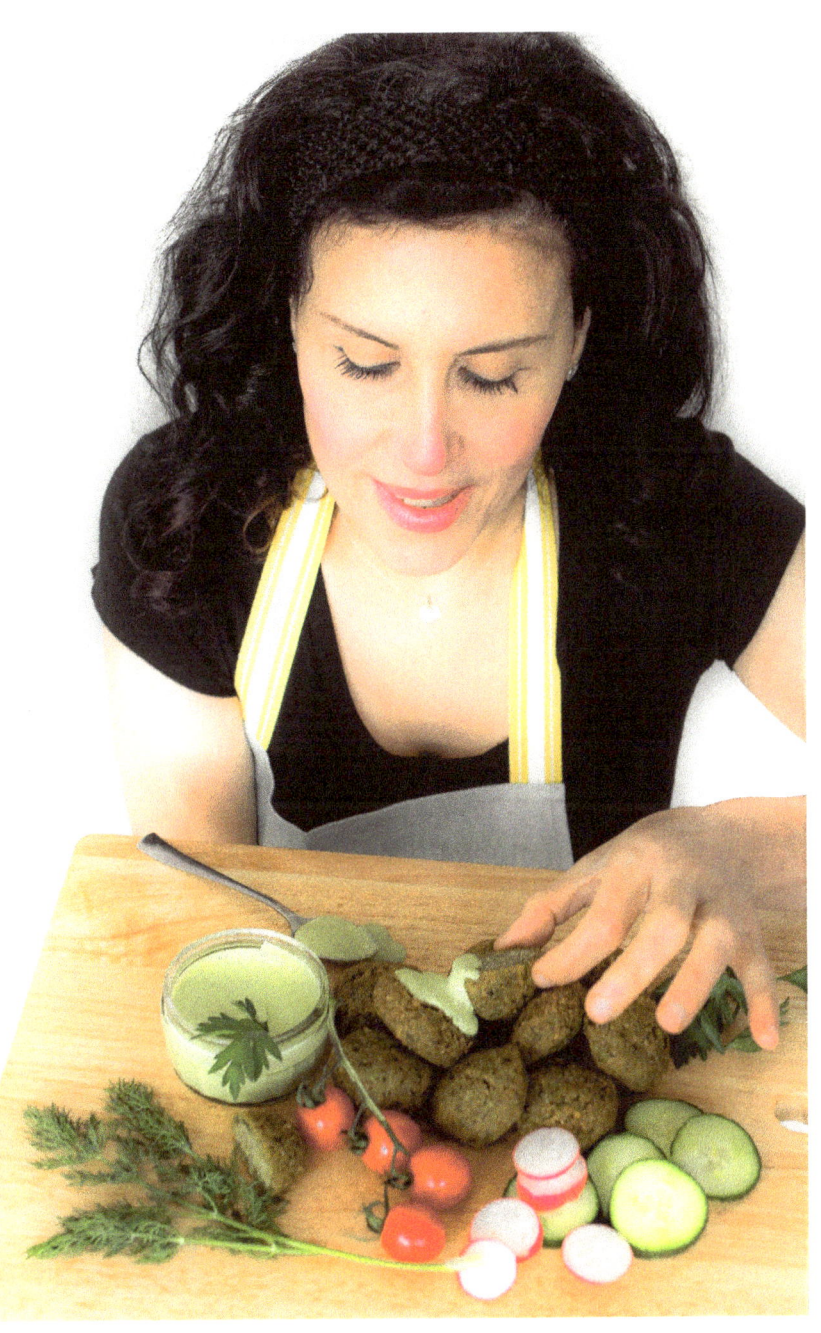

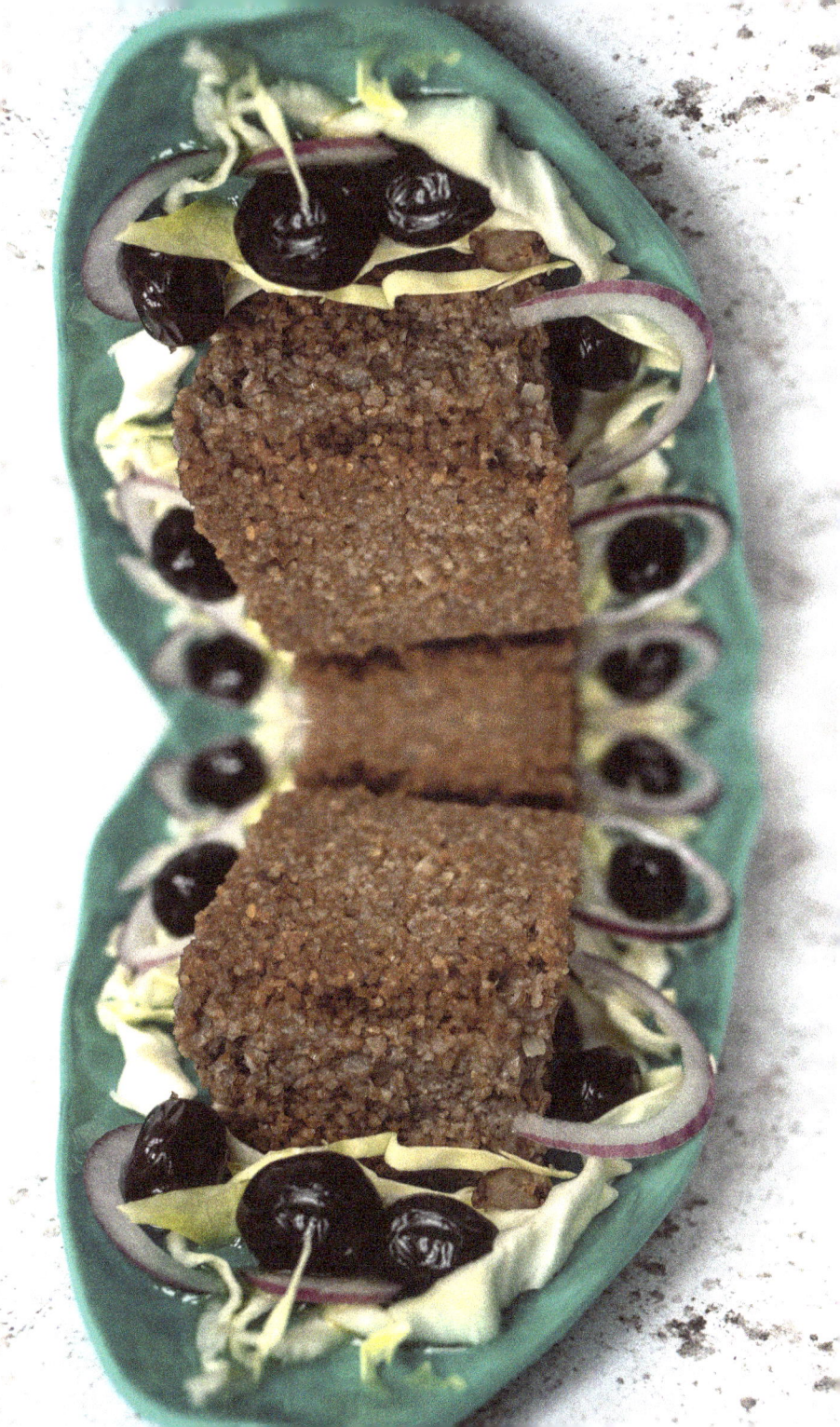

Contents

Introduction	xiv
My Life Through Food	xvii
Cooking Guide, Storage & Measurements	xx
Cooking Pulses	xxi
How to Store Herbs	xxv
Lentils	1
Okra with Red Lentil Dip	3
Mixed Lentil & Mushroom Soup	7
Bulgur	11
Bulgur with Green Lentils	13
Kibby Spices	17
Baked Bulgur Filled with Mushroom	19
Bulgur with Yoghurt & Cucumber	25

Contents

Beans	27
Cooking Stages	27
Mixed Beans	31
Chickpeas	35
Classic Hummus (Chickpea) Dip	37
Hummus with Crackers	41
Chickpea with Aubergine	45
Baked Cauliflower & Chickpea with Tahini & Peanut Butter Sauce	49
Chickpea with Bulgur	53
Fava/Broad Beans	55
Fava Bean & Chickpea Dip	57
Skinless Fava Bean with Dry Mallow Dip	61
Skinless Fava Bean with Peanut Butter Pâte	65

Contents

Dried Peas	69
Falafel Spices	71
Baked or Fried Pea Falafel with Tahini Sauce	73
Tahini Sauce	77
Quinoa	79
Dried Peas with Quinoa	81
Kabsa Spices	85
Freekeh	87
Freekeh with Mixed Nuts	89
Vine Wraps Stuffed with Freekeh & Herbs	93
Stuffed Aubergines & Courgettes in Tomato Sauce	97
Cabbage Wraps	101
Barley	105
Baked Vegan Burgers	107
Barley with Lentil & Crunchy Peanut Butter	111
Soya Mince	115
Grilled Vegan Kafta	117

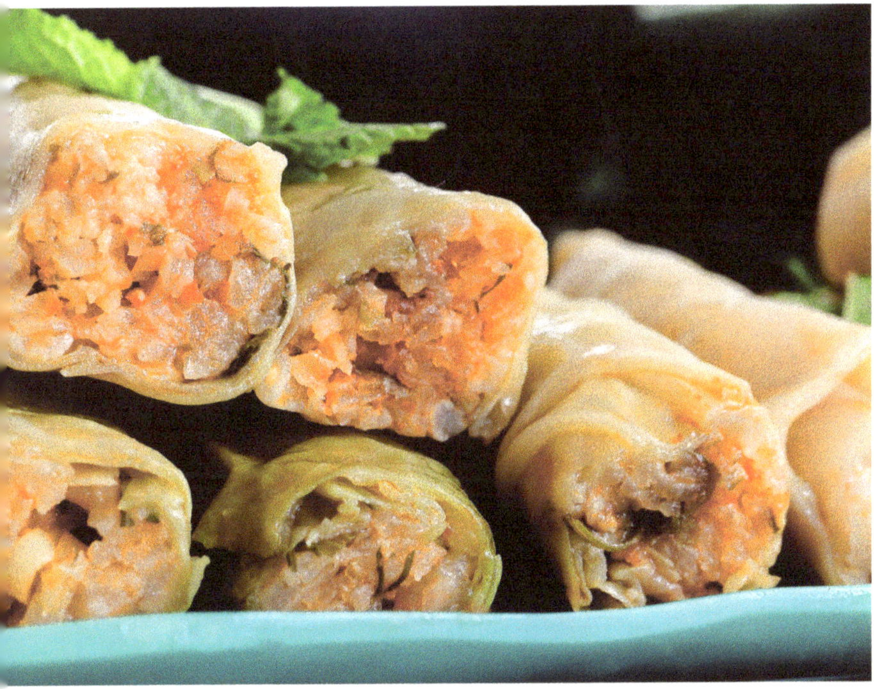

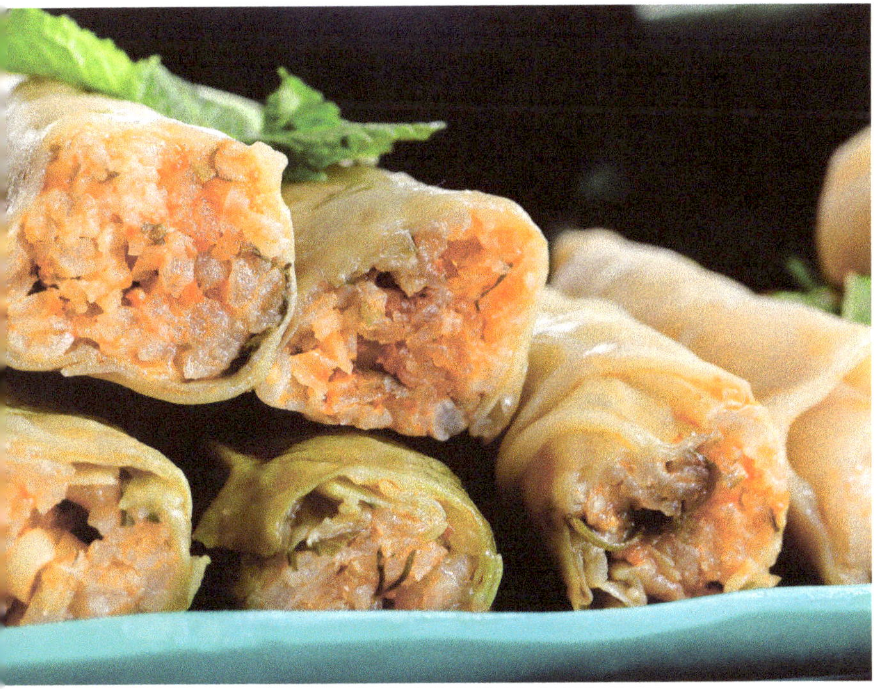

Introduction

This cookery book has been designed as a hand in developing your cooking skills and to make cooking easy, simple and enjoyable. The recipes in this book include the popular middle eastern herbs, seasoning and spices. These recipes also offer alternative ingredients to cater to individuals who are diabetic or have gluten intolerance, for example, exchanging wheat or bulgur with rice or beans.

In addition to learning how to cook delicious dishes, this book provides you with the understanding of basic cooking techniques that influence rich nutrients and flavors whilst eliminating the effects of compounds that reduce the bio availability of nutrients, including bloating and stomach discomfort. For instance, soaking pulses and discarding the water will weaken and reduce the phytate/phytic acid which binds/chelates to certain important minerals such as iron and prevents its absorption.

During my work I was surprised to find many individuals were unaware of how to cook pulses and grains from scratch. Pulses and grains are affordable and are a sustainable protein source, rich in soluble and insoluble fibre, complex carbohydrates, folate and vitamins. Additionally, they contain essential minerals such as magnesium, iron, potassium, zinc and calcium.

These recipes include a combination of pulses and grains to get the most out of the essential amino acids/protein that our bodies are unable to produce naturally.

Readers are welcome to ask questions or find out more about cooking techniques.

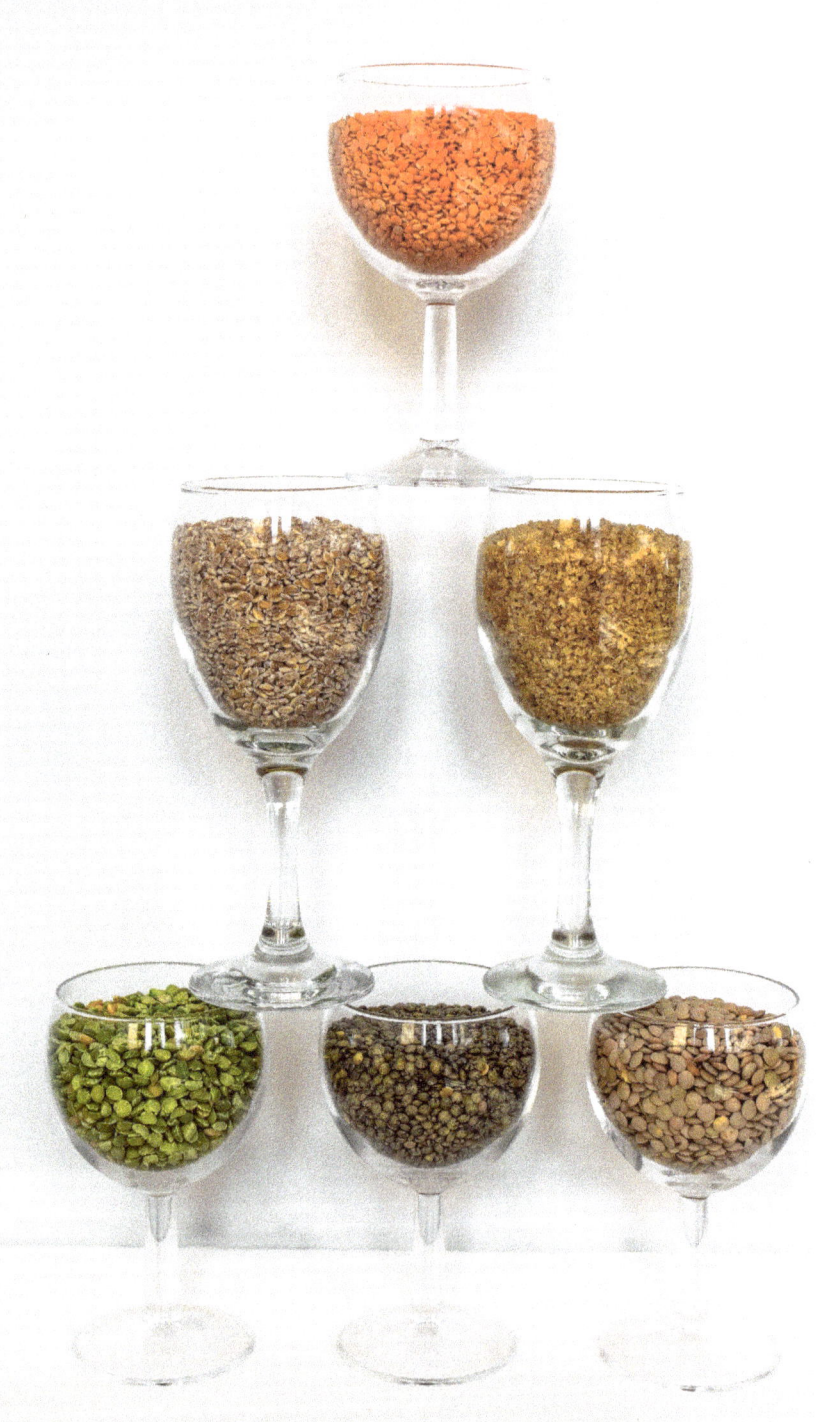

My Life Through Food

When reflecting on my childhood, I have certain memories that I cannot forget and once thought of, I am overcome by a warm nostalgia and appreciation for that fleeting period of our lives. Memories such as my first day at school, spending time on my kitchen floor helping my mother crack green olives with a wooden hammer and storing them in salty water. The smell of wild thyme when picking them on the mountains and of course, spending long summer days exploring our local area with my siblings and neighbours.

When we were hungry, we would alternate who's house we would have dinner at, and I clearly remember indulging ourselves in a variety of vegetarian foods. Foods such as wild malva parviflora and endivia which were cooked with olive oil and layered with rings of crunchy golden onions or freshly baked freekeh.

I look back on these days with great tenderness, for it has given me the appreciation I have today for cooking and healthy eating. My upbringing established my passion for selecting natural ingredients, preparing meals from scratch and creating tasty dishes and flavours. It created the foundations for my lifelong interest in food and so I went on to complete a bachelor's degree in Nutrition at university. Following this, I gained a postgraduate certificate in Clinical and Public Health Nutrition, where I was able to further understand the scientific elements of food and its effects on our health. I am now a proud member of the British Nutrition Association.

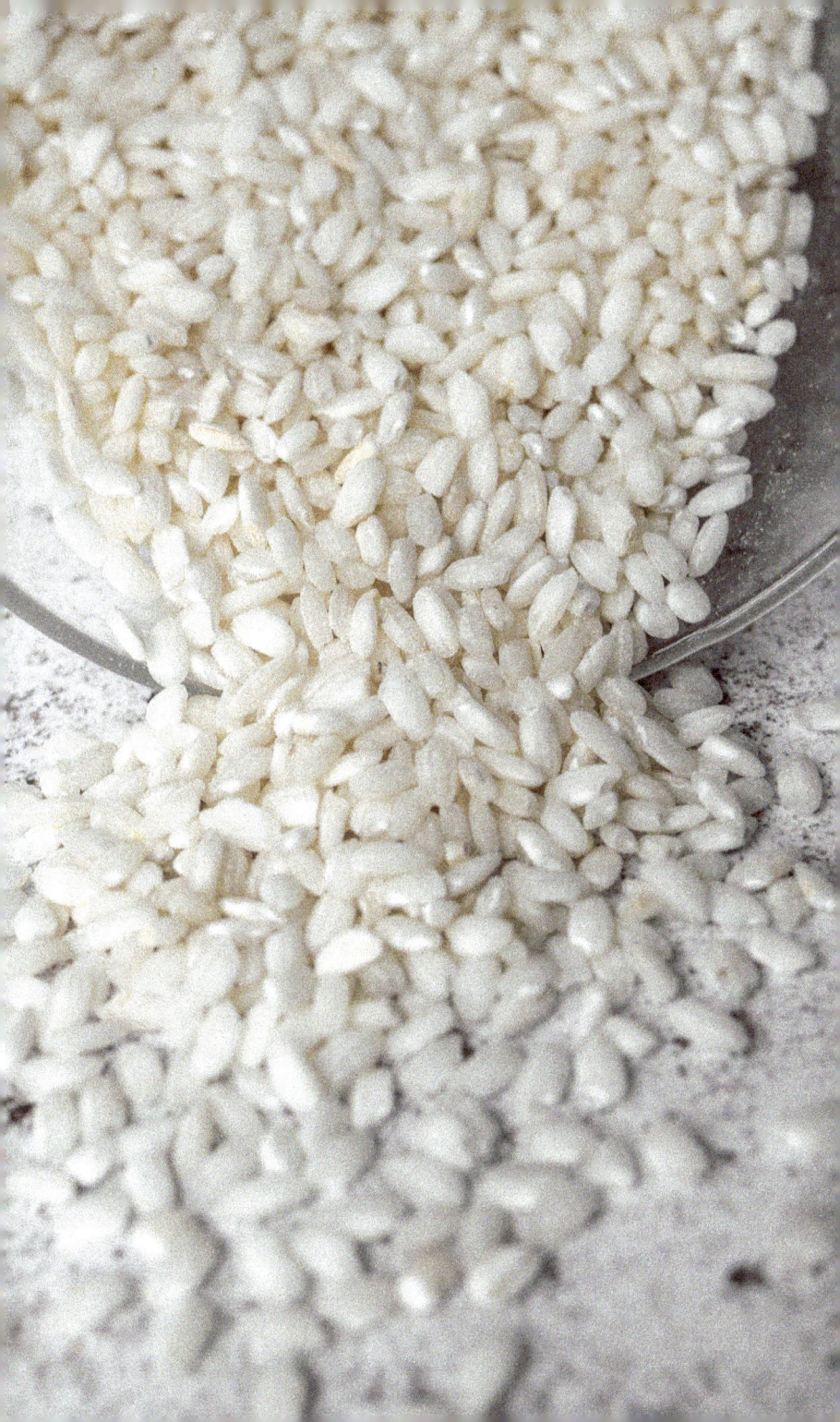

Cooking Guide, Storage & Measurements

- The main measurement used in my recipes is a 'cup' (approximately 240ml/8oz)
- The actual cooking time starts from the moment you reduce the heat after the food starts to boil. Slow cooking is essential in all pulses because it maximises the desired texture and flavour, whilst preserving the important nutrients. Additionally, cooking this way helps to prevent stomach upset and bloating. For individuals who suffer from bloating, add extra cumin powder to the pulses and 1/2-1 teaspoon of aniseed or fennel seed powder, depending on your taste.

Cooking Pulses

- Some pulses need to go through a primary cooking process before making a meal of them.

- They should be soaked in water overnight. Then drained and washed thoroughly, before placing in water to be boiled slowly.

- Add a teaspoon of baking soda to reduce the cooking time (optional). This may slightly modify the taste.

- Bring to boil and turn down the heat to let simmer slowly.

- Generally, all pulses take about 60-75 minutes to be cooked. Fava beans (with skin) will take about 4 hours.

- In the first stages of boiling, pulses tend to form a foam on the top of the saucepan. This foam needs to be collected with a spoon and discarded.

- After the pulses have finished boiling and have been drained, you can either use to cook right away with other ingredients to make a meal or separate them into meal sized portions, to be frozen and used at a later date. Only chickpeas and fava beans can be frozen in the water they were boiled in (stock). If you suffer from bloating, it may be better to drain the stock.

- Use chickpea or fava bean stock if they have been freshly boiled at home. If you are using cans, add boiled water instead.

- After cooking a meal, any leftovers can be cooled down and stored in the fridge. This will last about three days. In my opinion, all pulses taste more delicious the day after cooking.

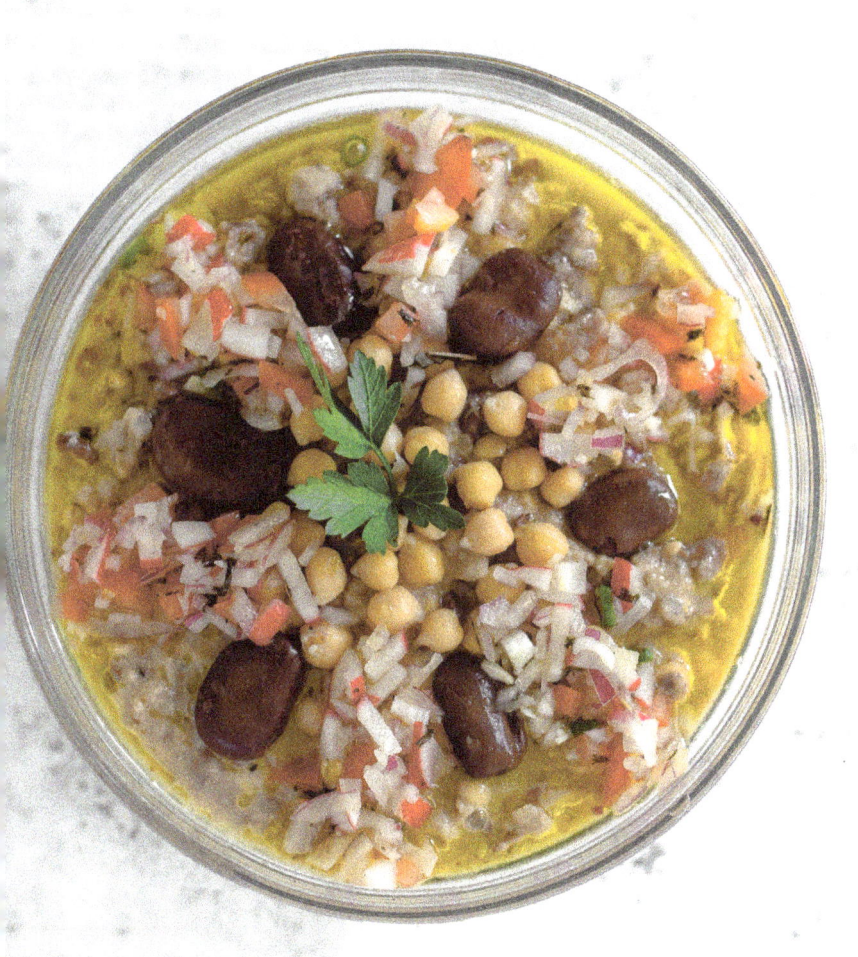

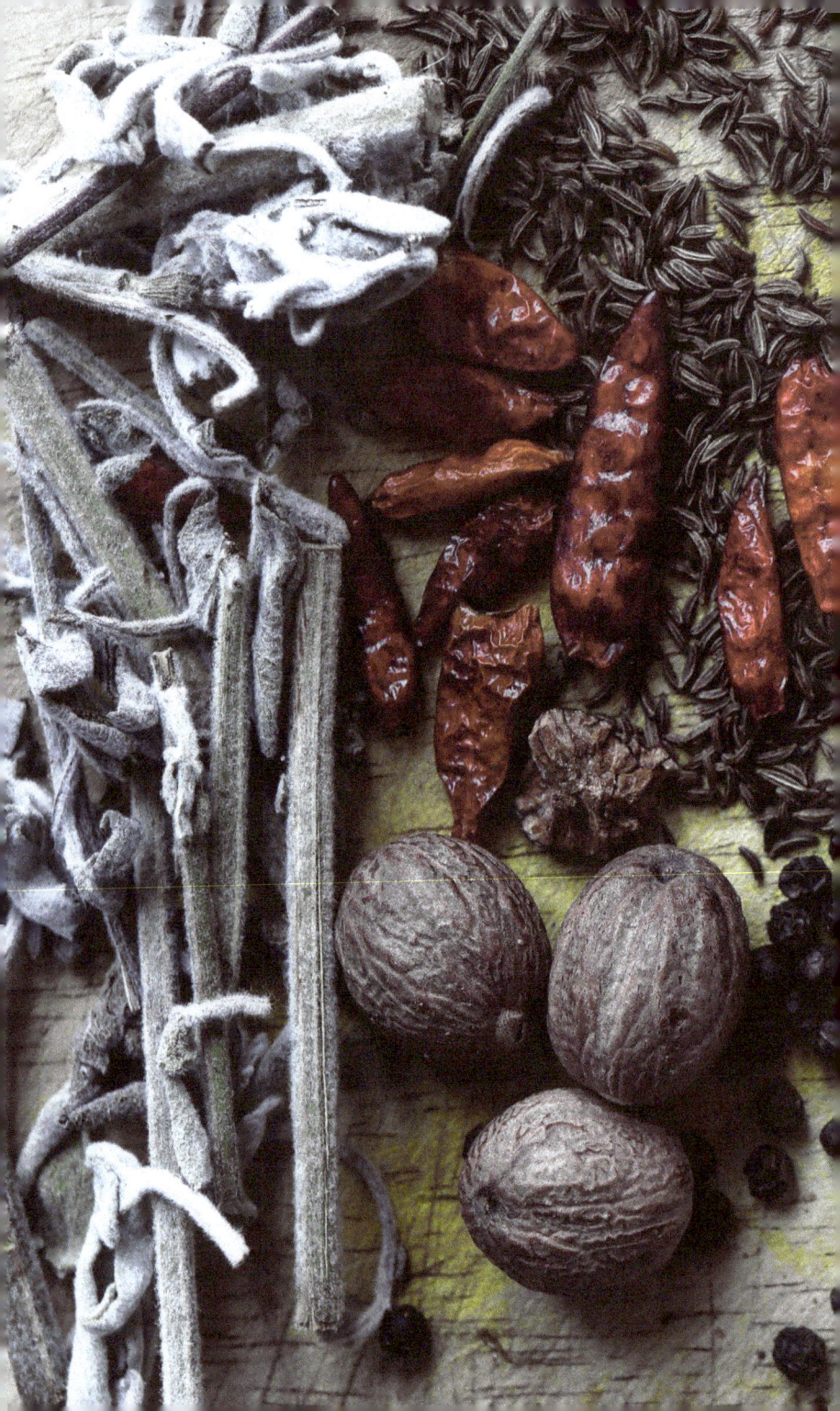

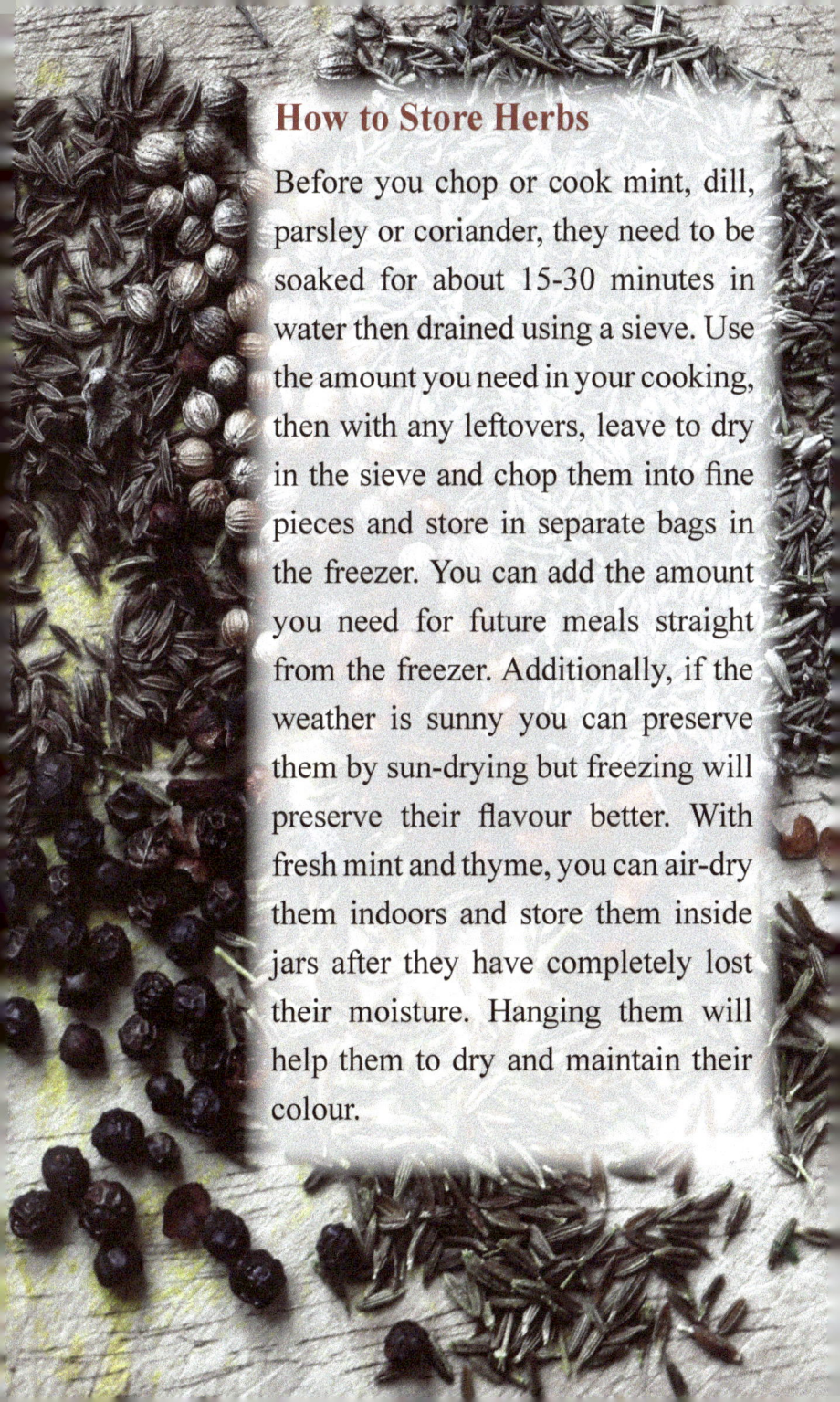

How to Store Herbs

Before you chop or cook mint, dill, parsley or coriander, they need to be soaked for about 15-30 minutes in water then drained using a sieve. Use the amount you need in your cooking, then with any leftovers, leave to dry in the sieve and chop them into fine pieces and store in separate bags in the freezer. You can add the amount you need for future meals straight from the freezer. Additionally, if the weather is sunny you can preserve them by sun-drying but freezing will preserve their flavour better. With fresh mint and thyme, you can air-dry them indoors and store them inside jars after they have completely lost their moisture. Hanging them will help them to dry and maintain their colour.

Lentils

Lentils do not need to be soaked in water the same way as other pulses, however you can soak them for an hour and discard the water before cooking to avoid bloating.

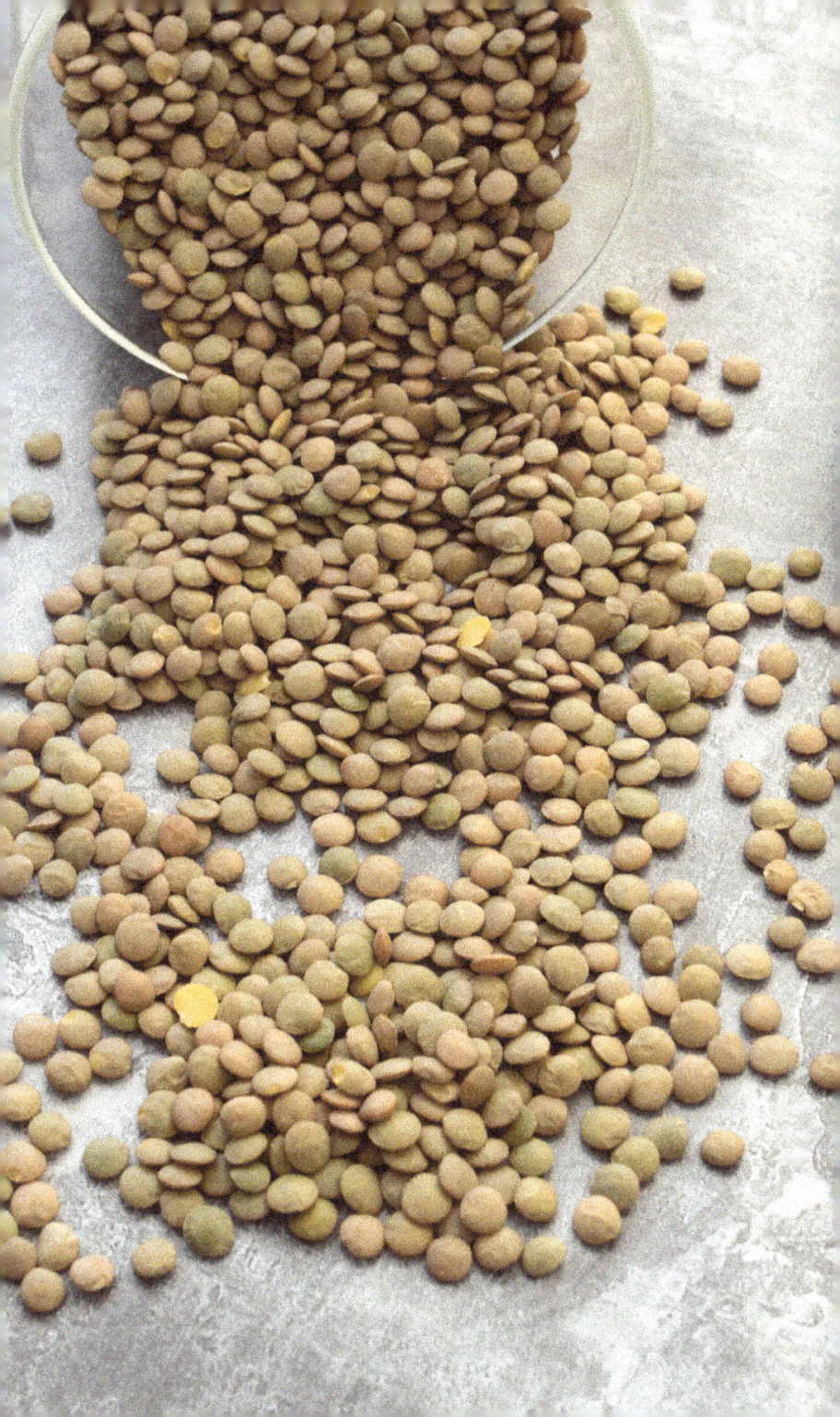

Okra with Red Lentil Dip

Ingredients

    1 cup dried red lentils

    200g grilled okra

    1 finely chopped onion

    3 cloves crushed garlic

    1 ¼ tsp sea salt

    ¼ cup olive oil

    ½ tsp cumin seeds

    ½ tsp cumin powder

    3 cups water

    ½ squeezed lemon juice

    1 chopped green chili (optional)

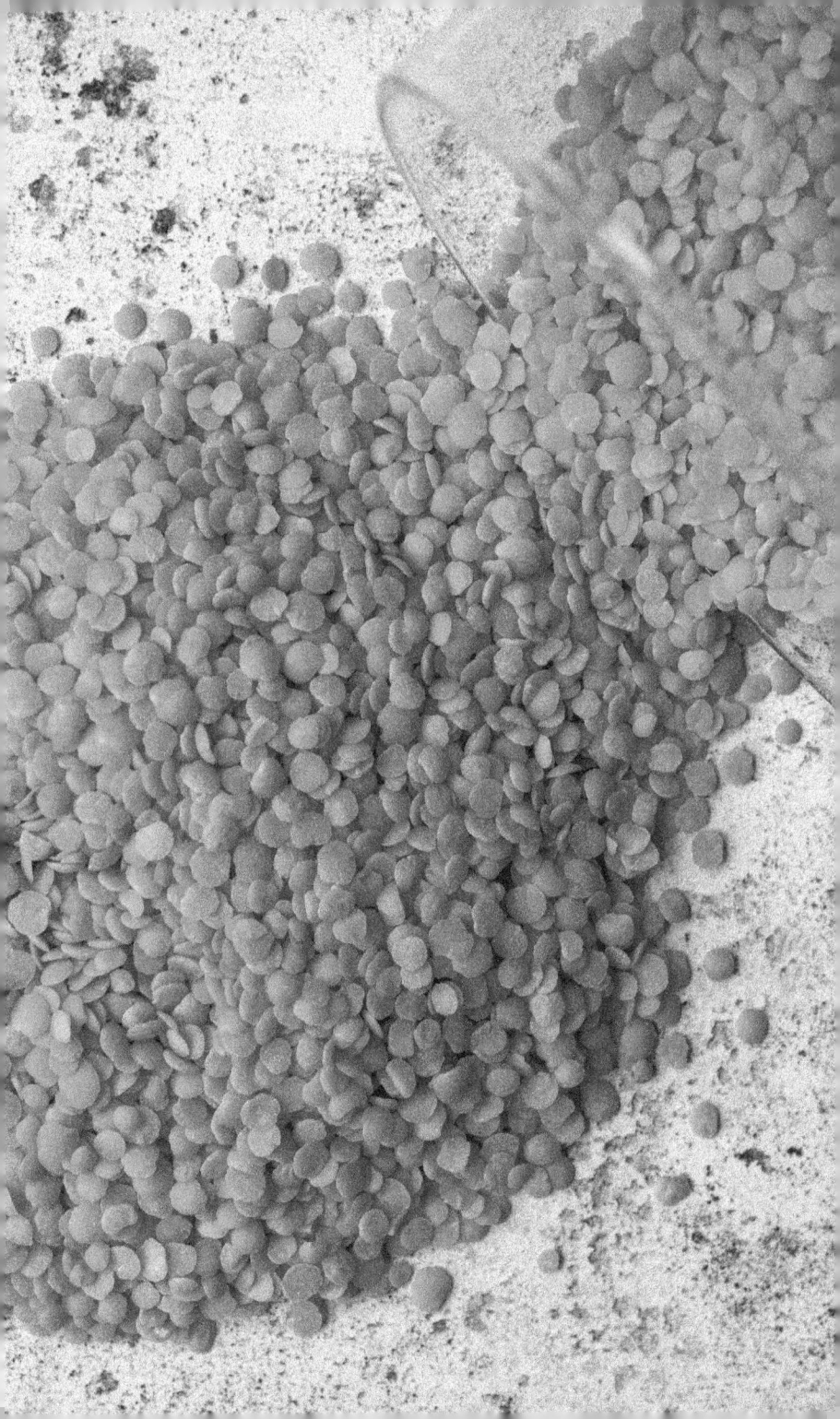

Preparation and Method

Remove the tops of the okra. Brush the okra with 2 tbsp of olive oil, then grill on both sides for about 7-10 minutes. Use a sieve to wash the lentils under hot water. Add 3 tbsp of olive oil to the saucepan, bring to a warm temperature then add the crushed garlic, onion, cumin seeds, green chili and sauté for 1 minute. Then add the water, cumin powder and salt. Finally, add the lentils with grilled okra, bring to boil, then reduce the heat and leave to simmer for about 1 hour.

After 1 hour increase the heat to just below medium and stir the mixture slowly whilst avoiding mashing the okra. Cover and leave for another 10-15 minutes.

Note: If you do not like okra, do not add and keep as a lentil dip. Serves 2. Serve with pitta bread or toast.

Tip: Delicious with radish.

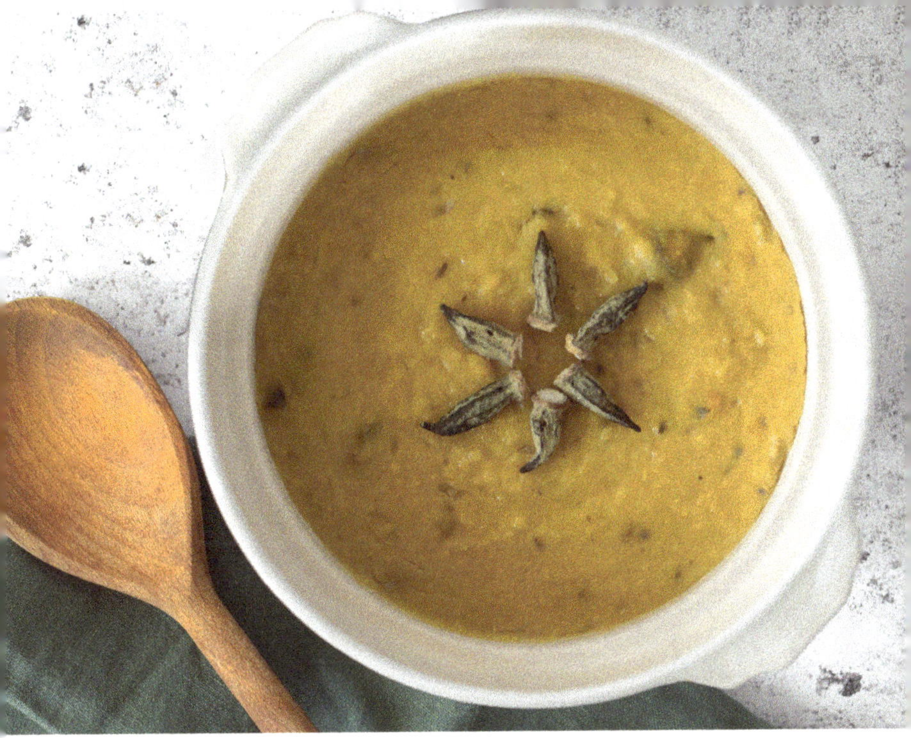

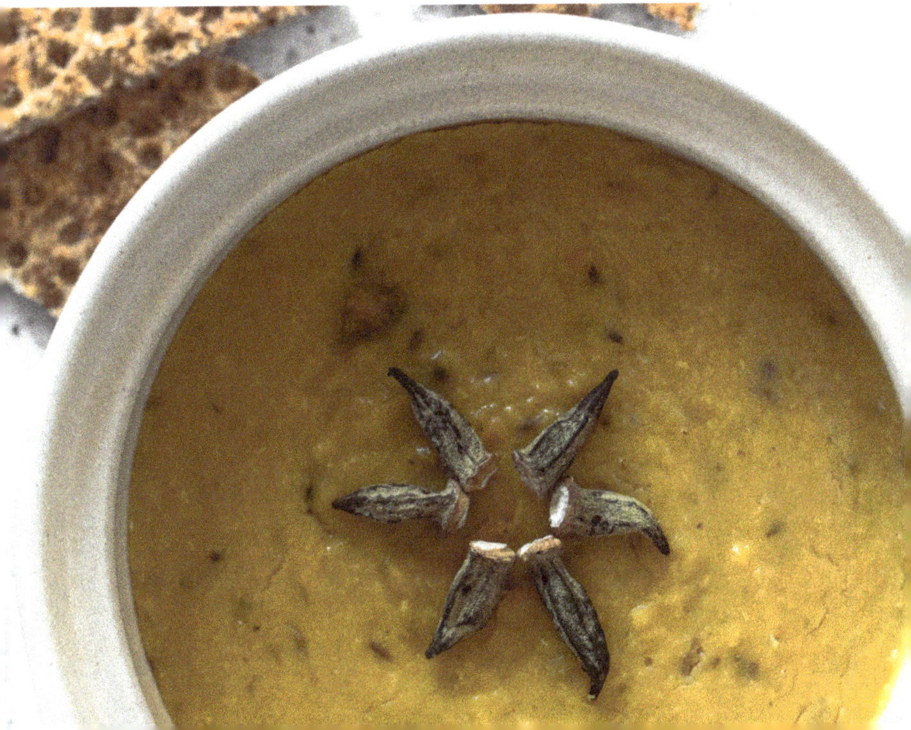

Mixed Lentil & Mushroom Soup

Ingredients

1 ½ cups dried red lentils

½ cup dried puy/ Canadian green lentils

500g chestnut mushrooms

1/3 cup olive oil (ideally extra virgin)

2 onions finely chopped

6 cups water

1 lemon or lime juice

2 tsp sea salt

2 tsp cumin powder

1 tbsp dry thyme

Thumb size finely chopped ginger

Cooking time 60-75 minutes.

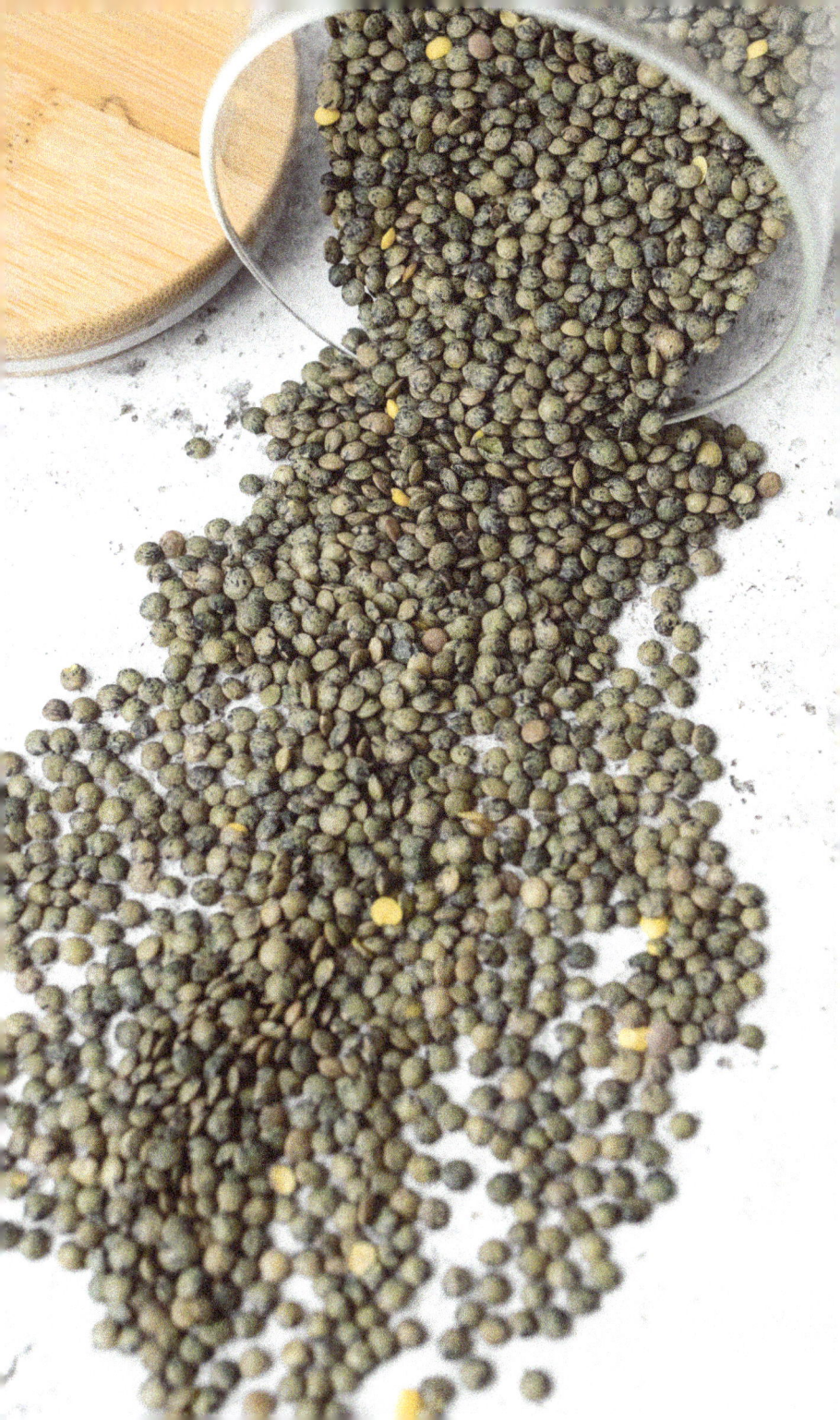

Preparation and Method

Wash the mixed lentils in a sieve, then add to the water in a saucepan and add cumin powder and salt. Once it starts to boil, reduce the heat and leave to simmer. Cut the mushrooms into slices and sauté them with a dash of olive oil and a pinch of salt for 1 minute or so, then add to the soup 15 minutes before the cooking time finishes.

Heat ¼ cup of olive oil in a pan and add the onion and ginger and stir until the mixture becomes a light golden colour and add to the saucepan of lentils.

In the last 15 minutes of the total cooking time, add the thyme and the remains of the olive oil to saucepan and cover with lid (not forgetting the mushrooms too). Finally, add the lemon or lime juice after you switch off the heat, before eating.

Tip: Nice to be eaten with dry bread or crackers.

Serves 2

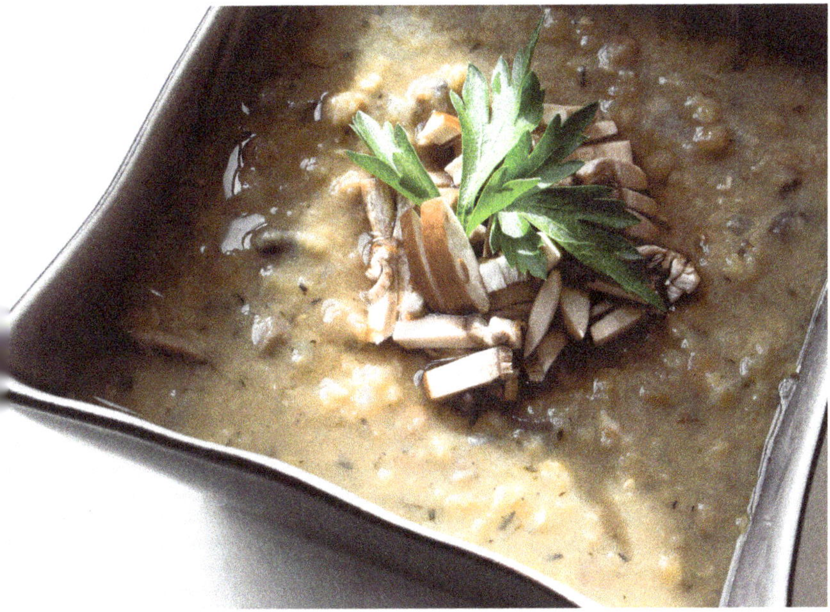

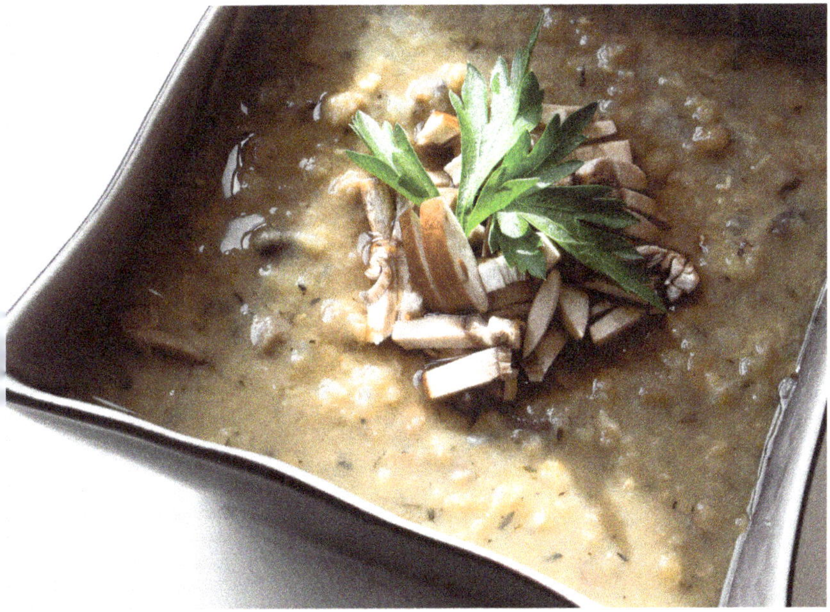

Bulgur

Bulgur (also known as Burghul) is a semi-boiled wheat and is made from different wheat families. It can come in different shades, sizes and colours and is high in fibre, protein and minerals in comparison to rice. Bulgur is easy to cook and can be mixed with other pulses and rice. It is used in many traditional recipes in middle eastern/Levantine cuisine.

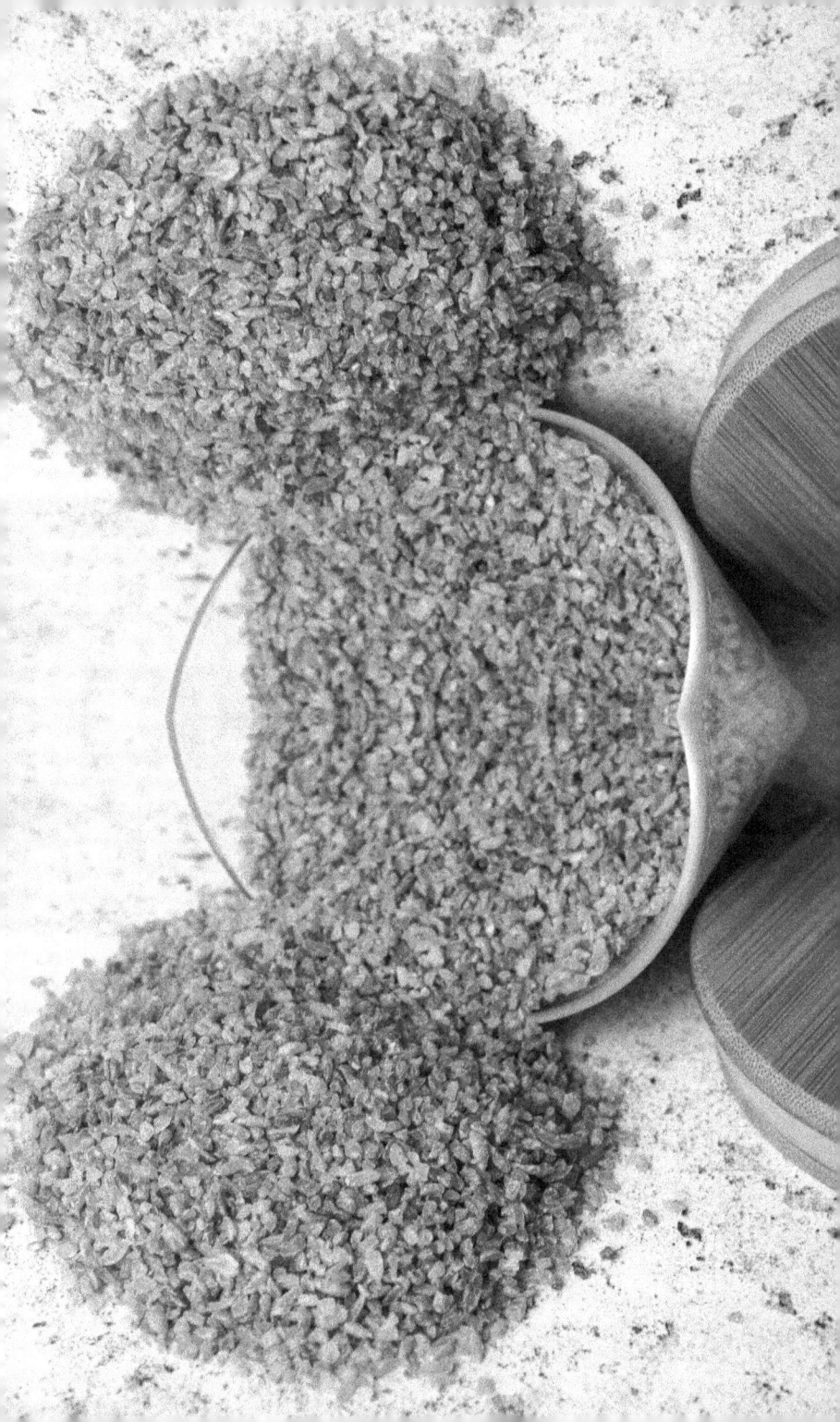

Bulgur with Green Lentils

Ingredients

    1 ½ cups dried green lentils

    1 cup coarse bulgur wheat

    2 chopped onions (medium size)

    2 tsp sea salt

    ½ tsp cinnamon

    1 tsp cumin powder & 1 tsp cumin seed

    1 ½ tsp garam masala

    ½ cup extra virgin olive oil

    4 cups water

    ½ cup crispy fried onion (optional)

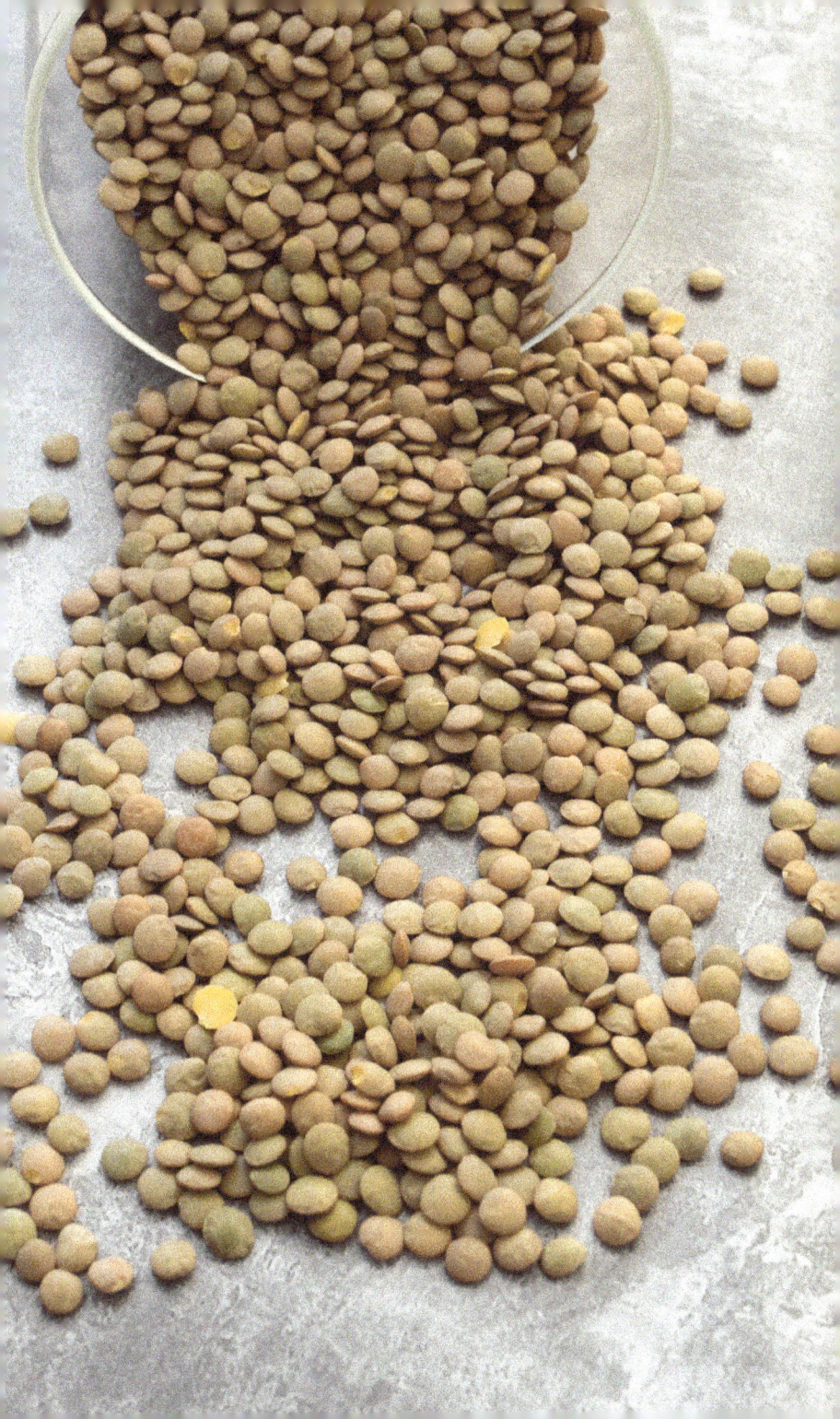

Preparation and Method

Wash the lentils in a sieve and add to the water in a saucepan, along with the bulgur. Add salt, cumin powder, cinnamon and gram masala. The moment it starts to boil, reduce the heat, cover with the lid and leave to simmer. Heat ¼ cup of olive oil in a pan with the onion and cumin seeds. Stir until they become a golden colour, then add to the saucepan. Stir and leave to cook in a very low heat for about 45-60 minutes. When finished, add ¼ cup of extra virgin olive oil, stir and leave to rest for 5 minutes before eating. Lastly, sprinkle crispy fried onion on top.

Tips: For the perfect meal, serve with tomato salad and vegan tzatziki. Alternatively, beetroot salad. Additionally, you can use the same ingredients to cook green lentils with rice.

Serves 4

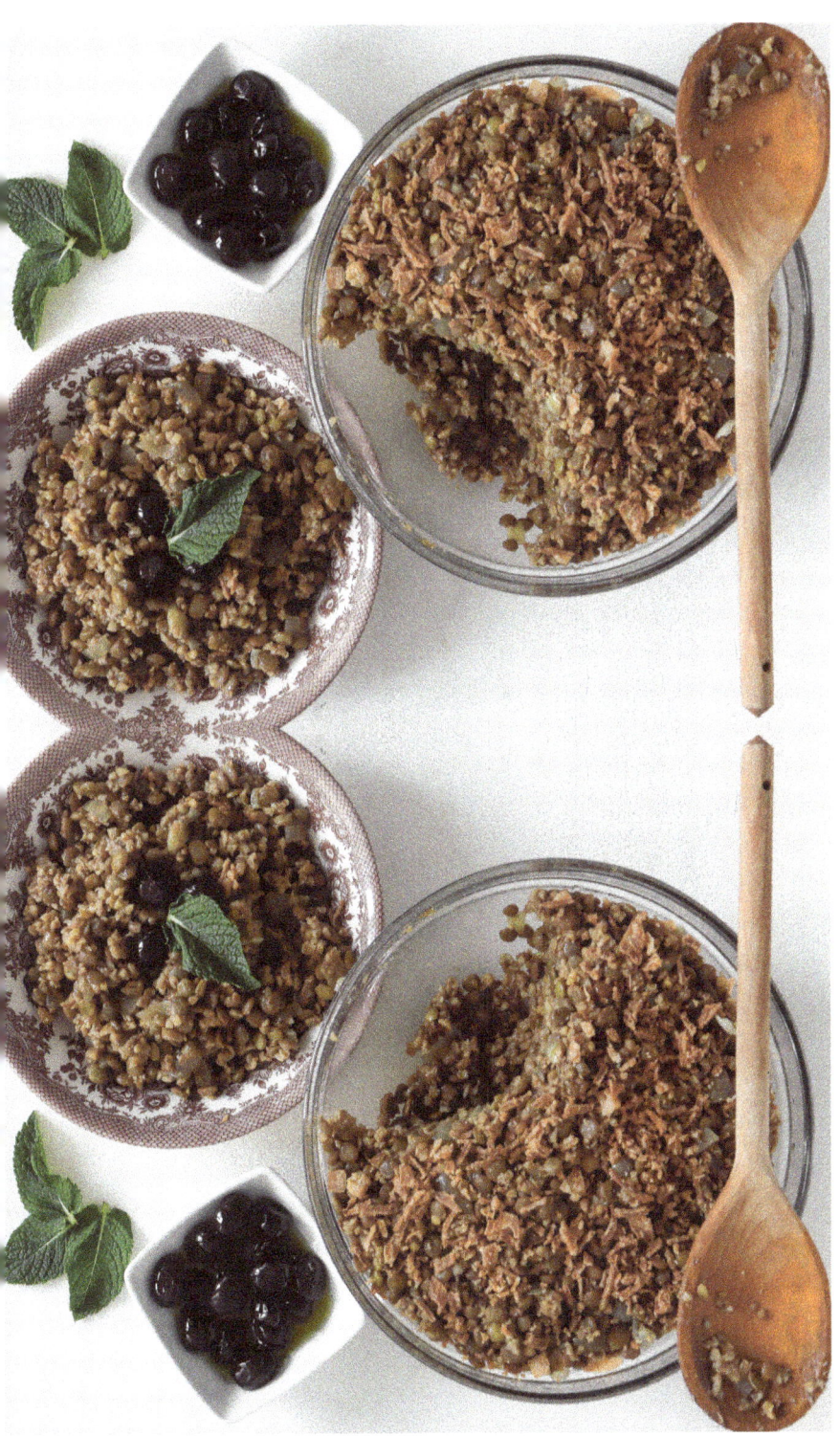

Kibby Spices

Ingredients

    1 tbsp dried rose leaves

    ¼ tbsp nutmeg

    ¼ tbsp black pepper

    ¼ tbsp marjoram

    ½ tsp red chili flakes

    ½ tsp paprika

    1 tbsp rosemary

    1 tbsp wild thyme

    1 tbsp cinnamon

    1 tbsp cumin

    1 tbsp basil

    1 tbsp dried mint

    2 cloves

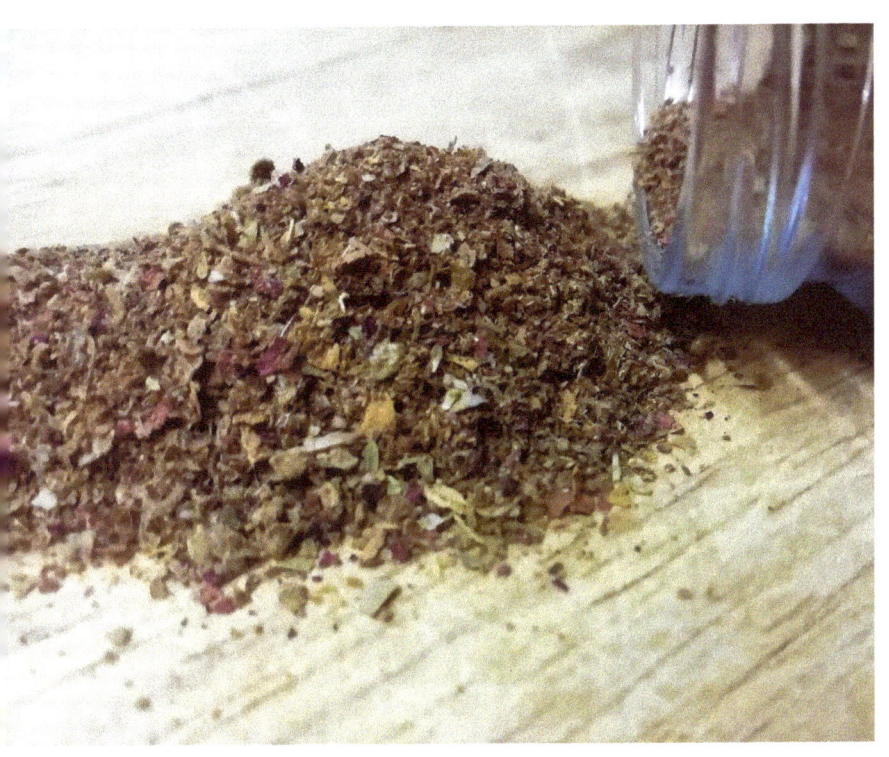

Tips: If you grind the spices before adding to the food, a lovely fragrance with be released along with a rich taste. It can also be ground and stored in a glass jar for later use. Alternatively, kibby spices are usually available to buy from middle eastern food stores.

Baked Bulgur Filled with Mushroom

Ingredients

   2 cups fine/small bulgur

   1 ½ cups water

   2 medium boiled potatoes

   500g chopped mushrooms

   ½ cup grated vegan mozzarella cheese

   2 small fine chopped onions

   3 crushed garlic cloves

   ½ cup olive oil

   2 ½ tsp sea salt

   2 ¼ tsp kibby spices

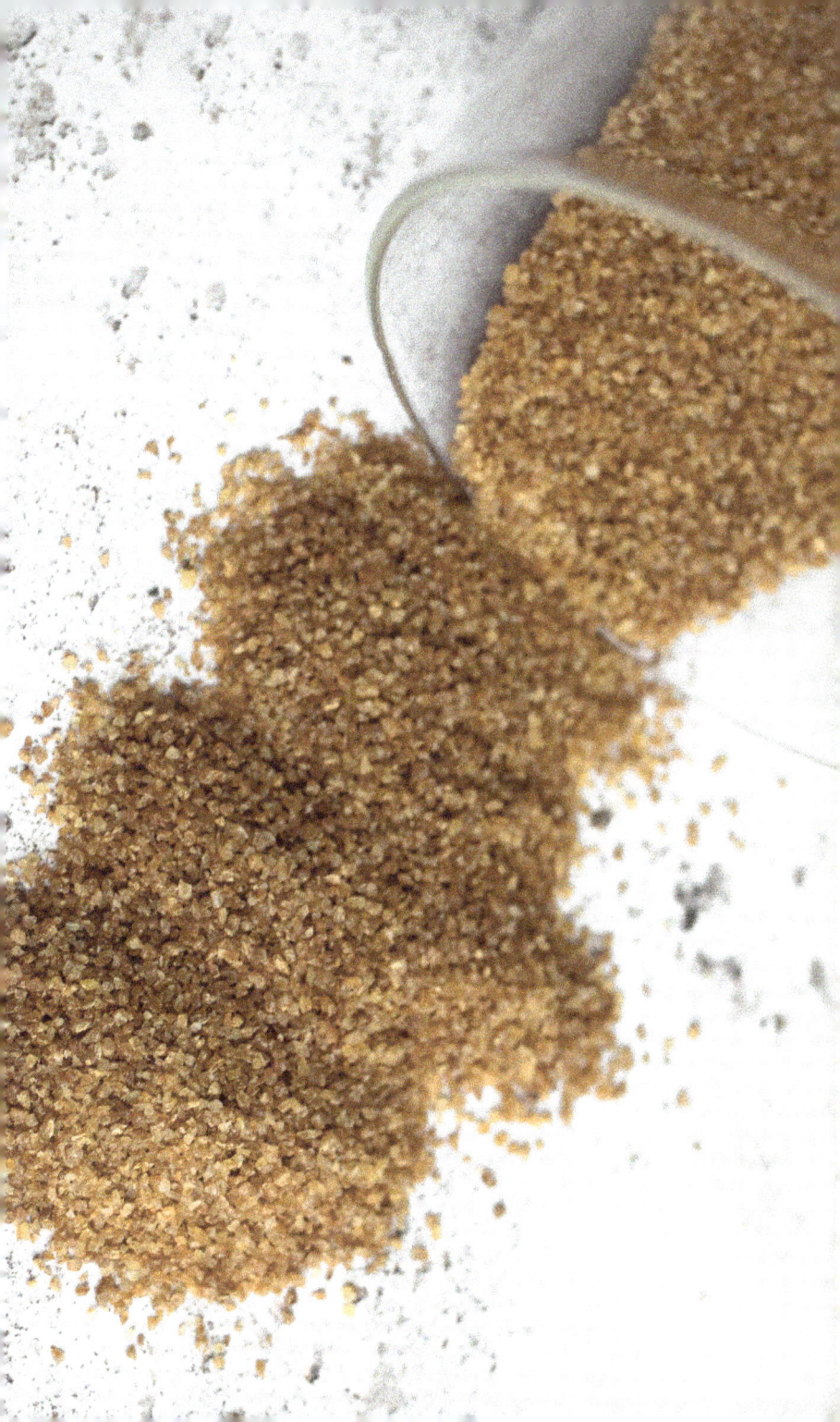

Preparation and Method

Soak the bulgur in 1½ cups of water for 1½ hours in a large bowl. Sauté the mushrooms with 1 onion in 3 tbsp of olive oil and ½ tsp of salt on a low to medium heat. Continue stirring for about 5-7 minutes or until mushroom stock is produced. Keep the stock aside to use later.

Mash the potatoes and add to the bulgur. Then add kibby spices, salt, onion, mushroom stock and the remaining olive oil. Knead the ingredients together until it becomes a dough-like consistency.

Divide the mixture into 2 sections. Brush a medium sized baking tray with oil and using one section of the mixture, spread one layer into the tray.

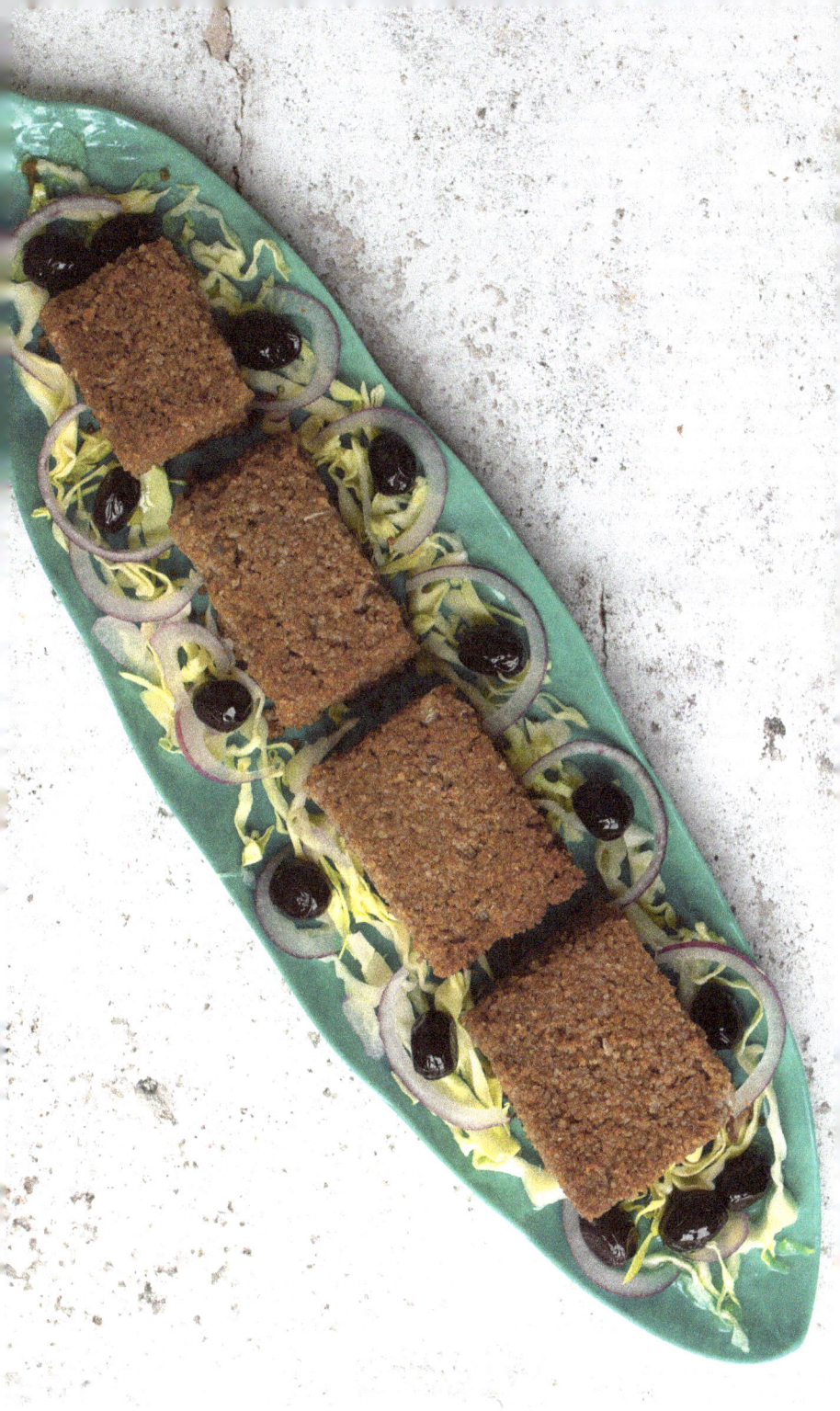

Next, spread the mushroom filling with the cheese on top of the layer and then carefully use the other section to layer the rest of mixture on top of the mushroom and cheese filling. To make sure the surface is even and smooth, wet both hands with water and gently smooth over the surface.

Finally, dress the top layer with a tbsp of olive oil by hand and then with a knife, cut into squares before placing it in the oven. Place in the middle of the oven after it has preheated to 200 degrees Celsius for 25 minutes. Once done leave for 5 minutes to rest.

Serves 4-5

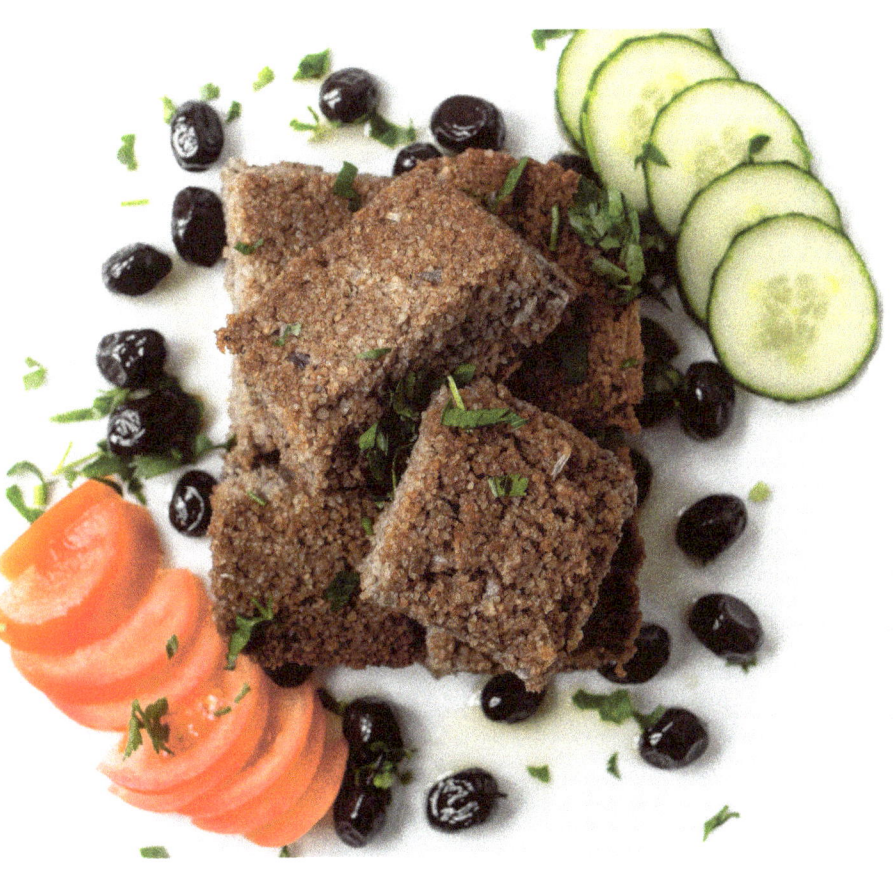

Bulgur with Yoghurt & Cucumber

Ingredients

    1 cup sugar free soya yoghurt

    ½ cup coarse bulgur

    ¼ cucumber chopped into slim slices and quartered

    ½ tsp sea salt

    1 crushed garlic clove

    1 tbsp olive oil

    1 tbsp dry mint

    1 ½ cups water

    Hand full of pine nuts

Preparation and method

Boil the bulgur in water for 10 minutes. Drain all the water completely with a sieve. Add the boiled bulgur, cucumber, mint, salt and olive oil to the soya yoghurt in a bowl. Scatter roasted pine nuts on top.

Serves 2

Tip: Alternatively, you can use sugar free coconut or almond yoghurt.

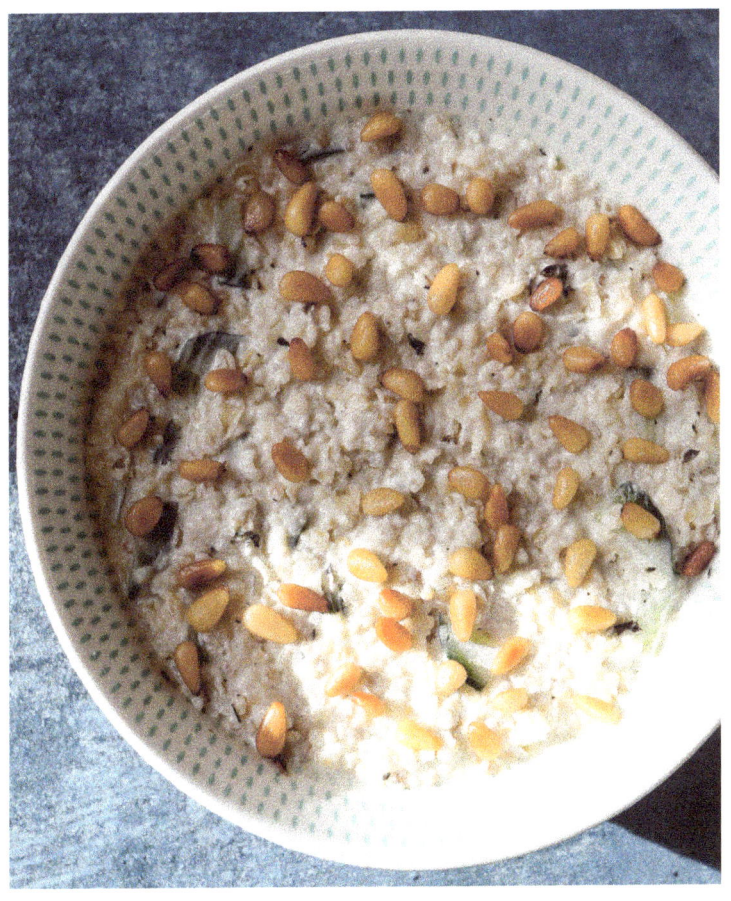

Beans

Cooking Stages

500g of dry pulses are about 1400g of cooked pulses (approximately 5 cans of cooked pulses), therefore buying dry pulses will save a lot of metal waste. Dry beans/pulses such as, chickpeas, fava beans, kidney beans, navy, black and rosecoco/ pinto beans, all need to go through a primary cooking process before making a meal of them.

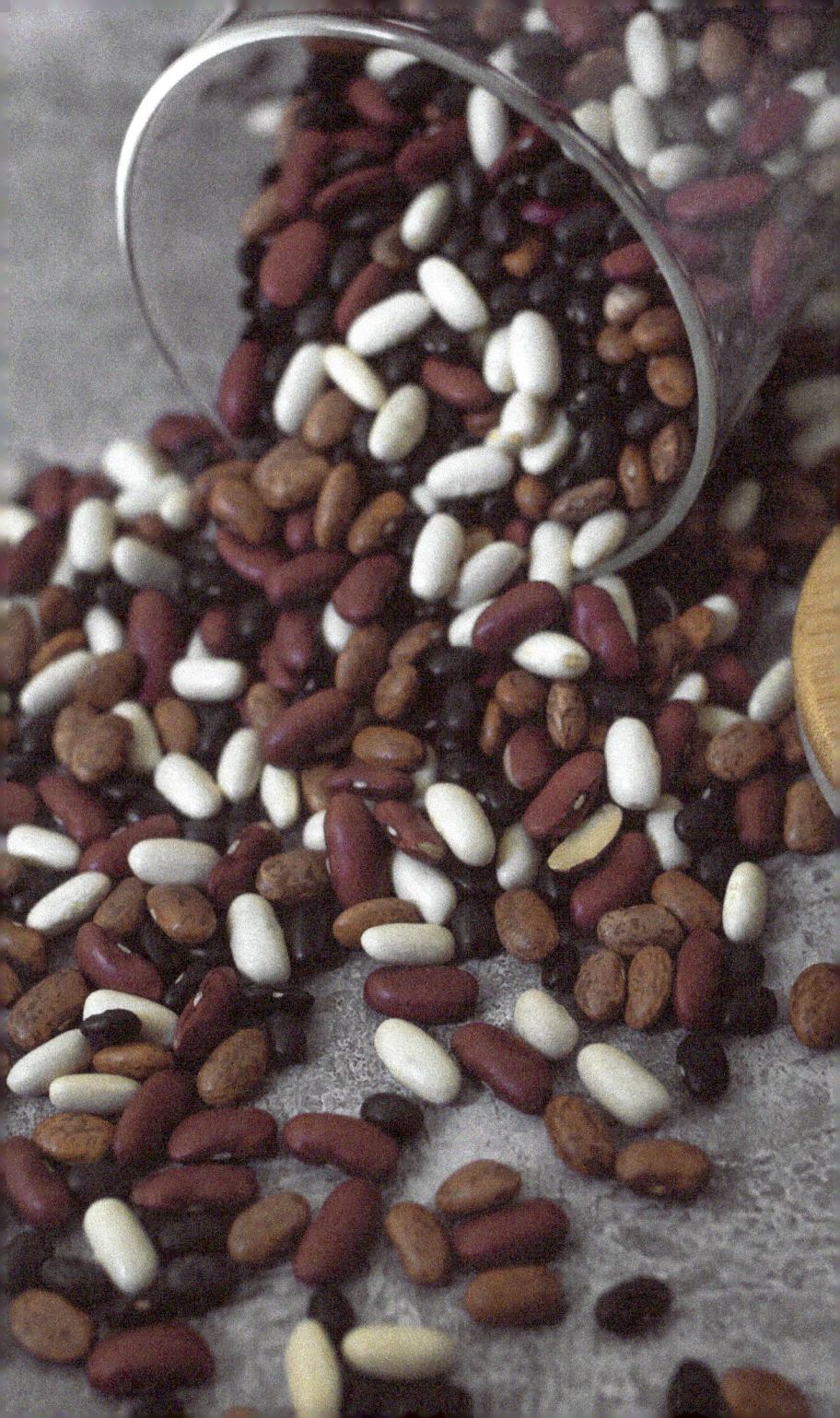

Wash and soak the total 500g of dry beans in plenty of water overnight. The following day, drain the water and wash them thoroughly. Then fill the saucepan with a generous amount of water, bring to boil then reduce the heat to allow to simmer slowly for 60-75 minutes. Once done, drain the water and wash them again. It is important to drain the cooking water to remove some of the unhealthy compounds that exist in some beans and to prevent bloating and gut discomfort that some people experience. At this stage they are ready to be cooked with other ingredients or divided into smaller amounts and stored in the freezer for future meals.

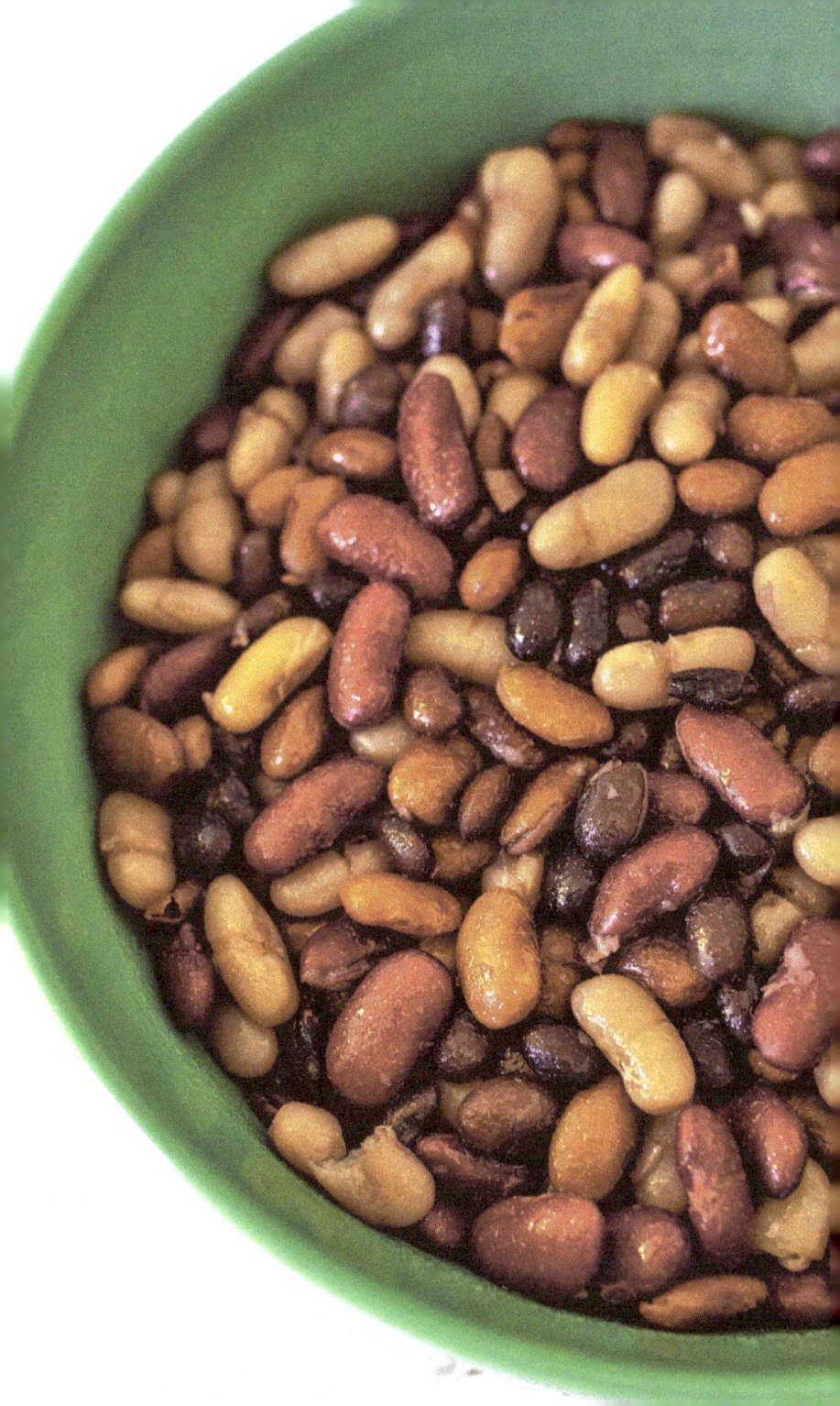

Mixed Beans

Ingredients

2 ½ cups dried mixed beans (soaked in water overnight)

2 large chopped onions

8 cloves crushed garlic

2 ½ tsp sea salt

2 tsp cumin powder

1 ½ tsp turmeric powder

2 thumb sized pieces of chopped ginger (50g)

1 lime/lemon juice

2 tbsp tomato puree

2 chopped tomatoes

1 cup extra virgin olive oil

2 cups boiled water

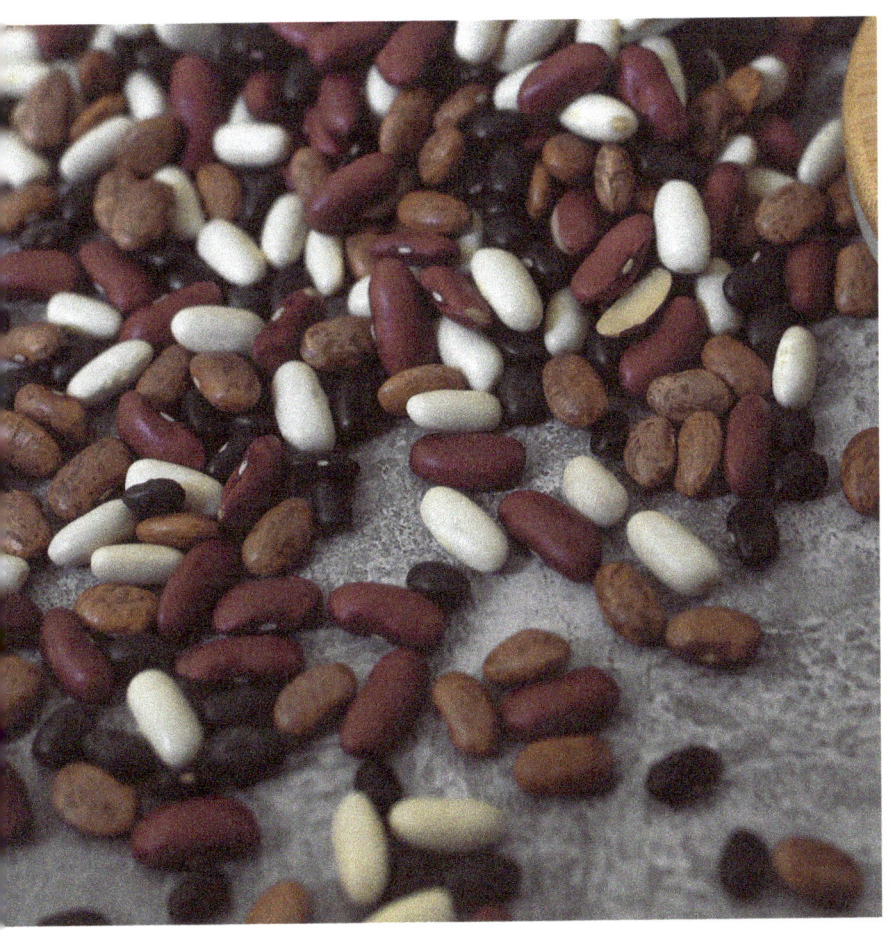

Preparation and Method

Note: After crushing the garlic, mix with a tbsp of olive oil and leave aside until needed.

Wash and soak the mixed beans in cold water overnight (this equates to roughly 4 shop bought cans). The next day, drain the water and rinse thoroughly.

Fill a saucepan with a generous amount of water, bring to boil then reduce heat to allow the beans to simmer slowly for 50-60 minutes. When done, drain the water, rinse again and put aside. Sauté the onion, ginger and half the amount of garlic in 3 tbsp of olive oil for 2 minutes. Add the tomatoes and stir for 2 minutes.

Add the beans, boiled water, olive oil, salt, cumin, turmeric and the tomato puree. When the mixture reaches boiling point, reduce the heat and leave to simmer for about 45 minutes. After turning the heat off, stir in the lime juice and the rest of the garlic. Leave to rest for 5 minutes before eating. Serve with boiled rice.

Serves 5-6

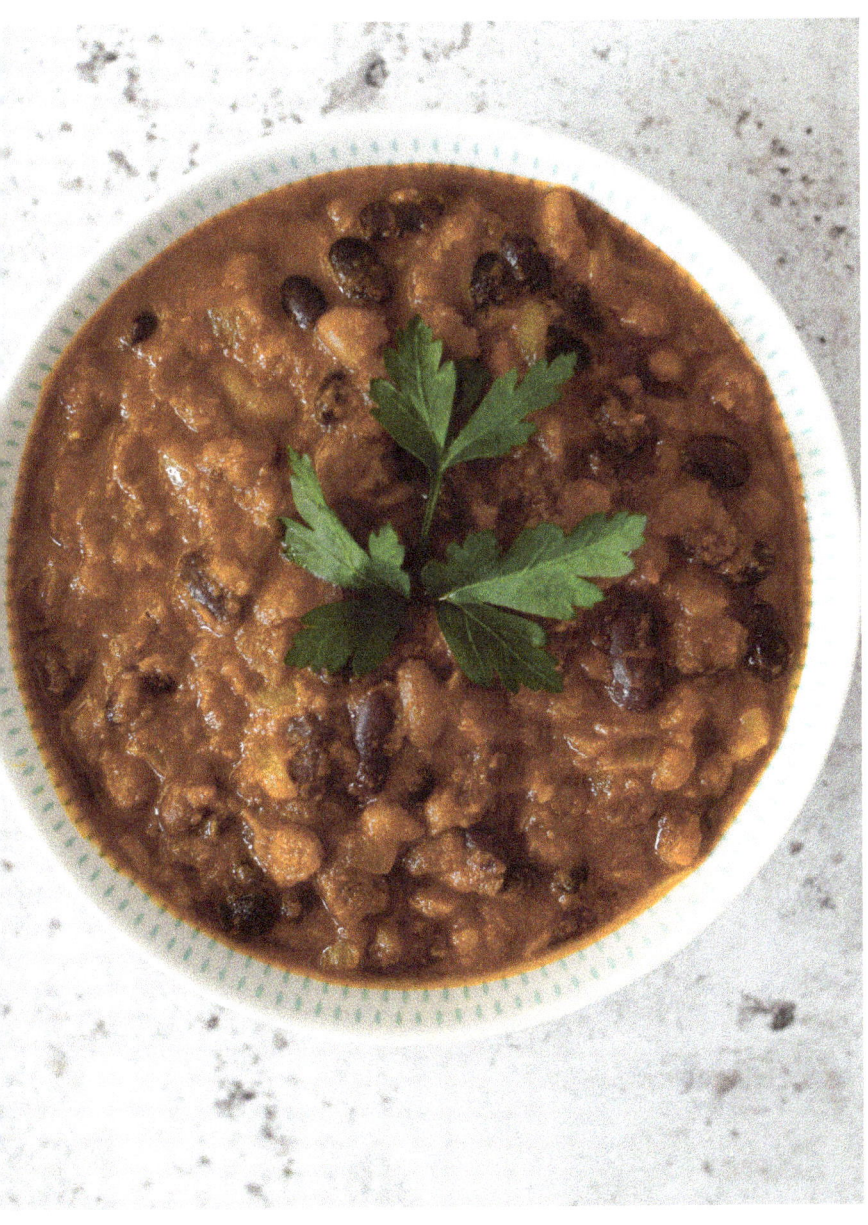

Chickpeas

Chickpeas are a form of legumes. In the middle east they are called 'hummus' and contain a high level of protein, vitamins, minerals, fat and soluble fibre.

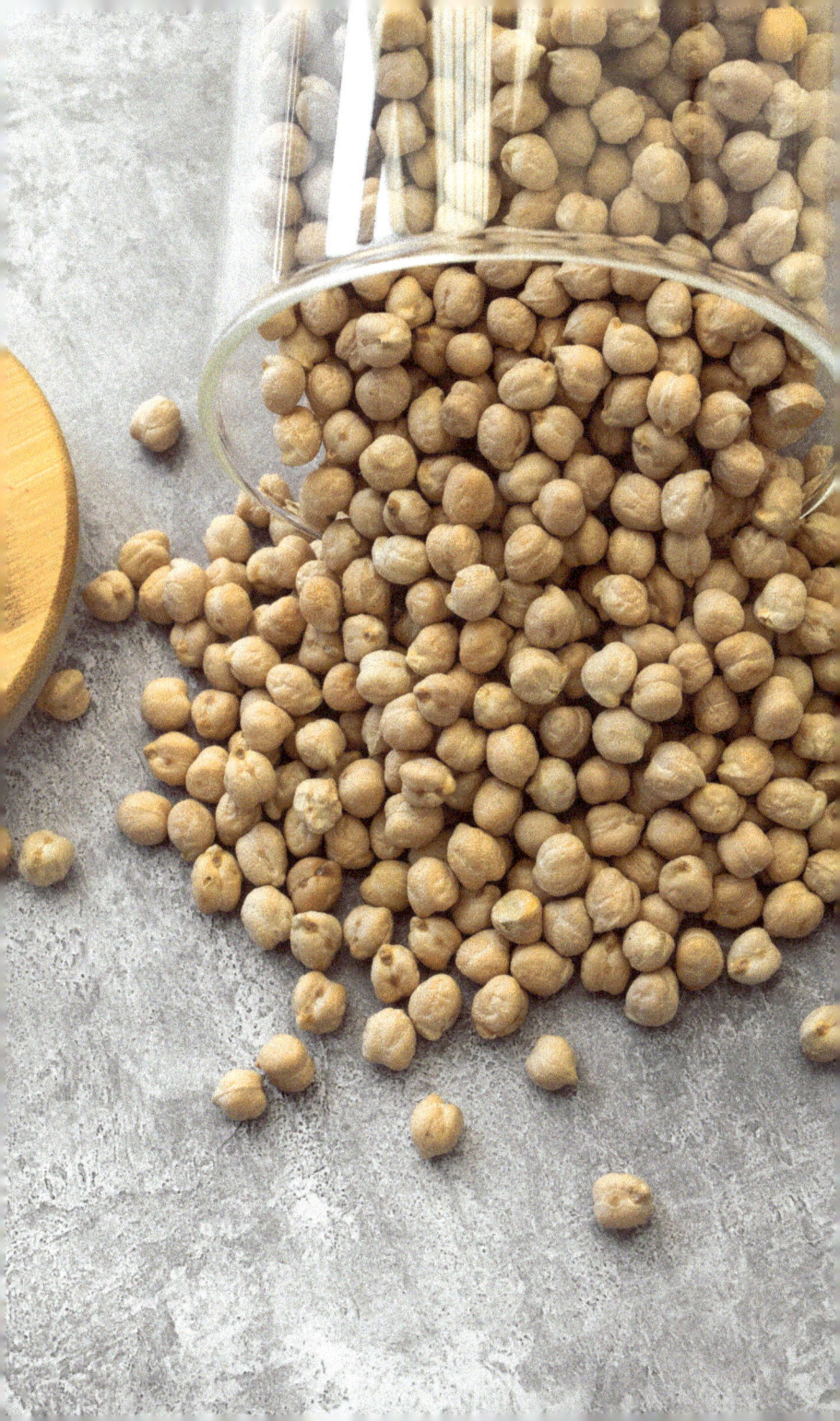

Classic Hummus (Chickpea) Dip

2 cups boiled chickpeas

2 tbsp tahini paste

1 lemon juice

1/3 cup hummus stock or water

1 ½ garlic cloves

½ tsp cumin Powder

1 ½ tsp sea salt

3 tbsp extra virgin olive oil

Red chili powder (for seasoning)

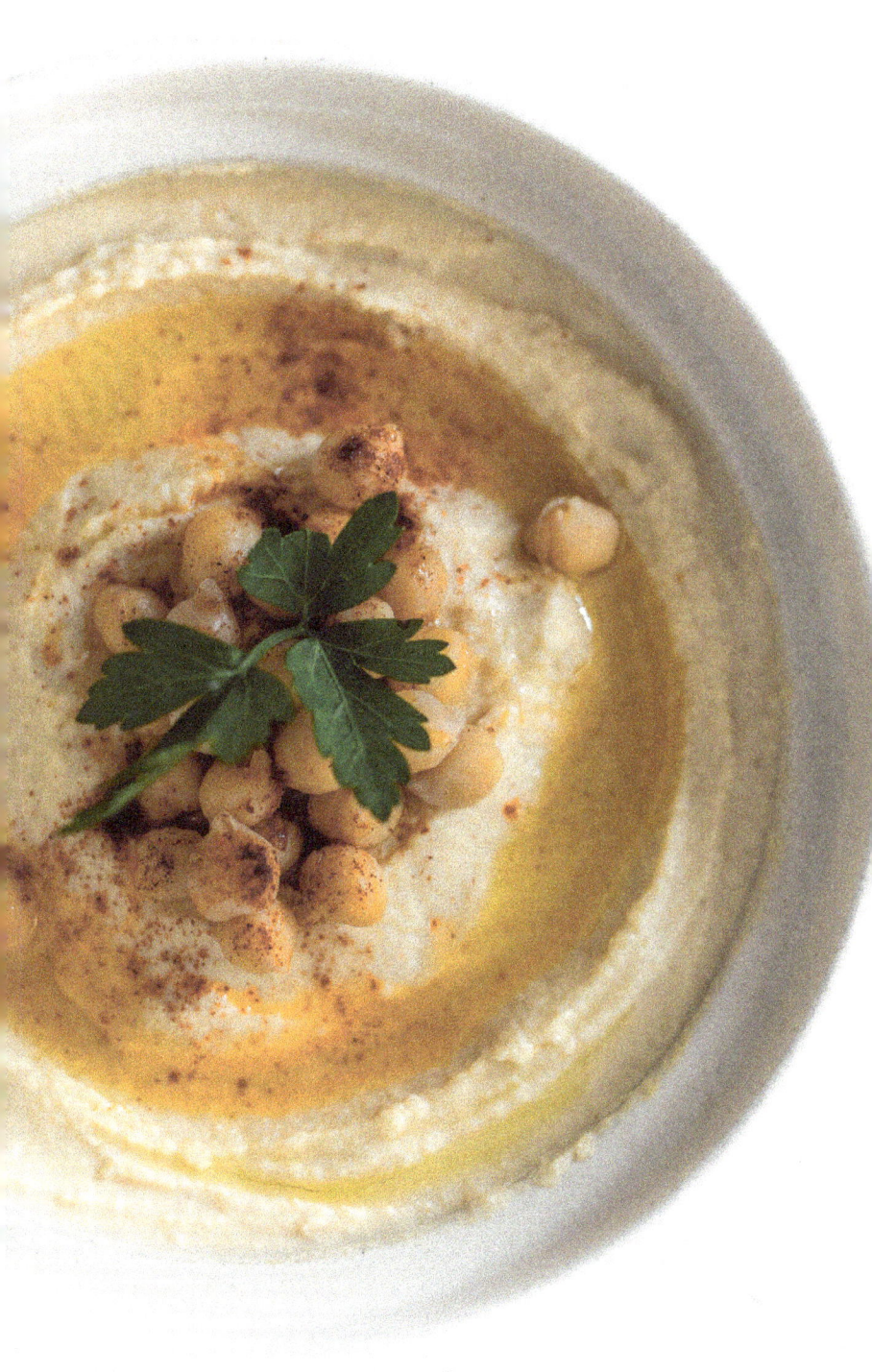

Preparation and Method

Blend all the ingredients in a mixer until smooth (if you do not have a mixer, use a potato masher). Empty hummus onto a plate and dress with olive oil and a sprinkle of red chili powder.

Serves 3-4

Tips: Top with roasted pine nuts or sumac instead of red chili powder. Additionally, you can use almond butter instead of tahini paste.

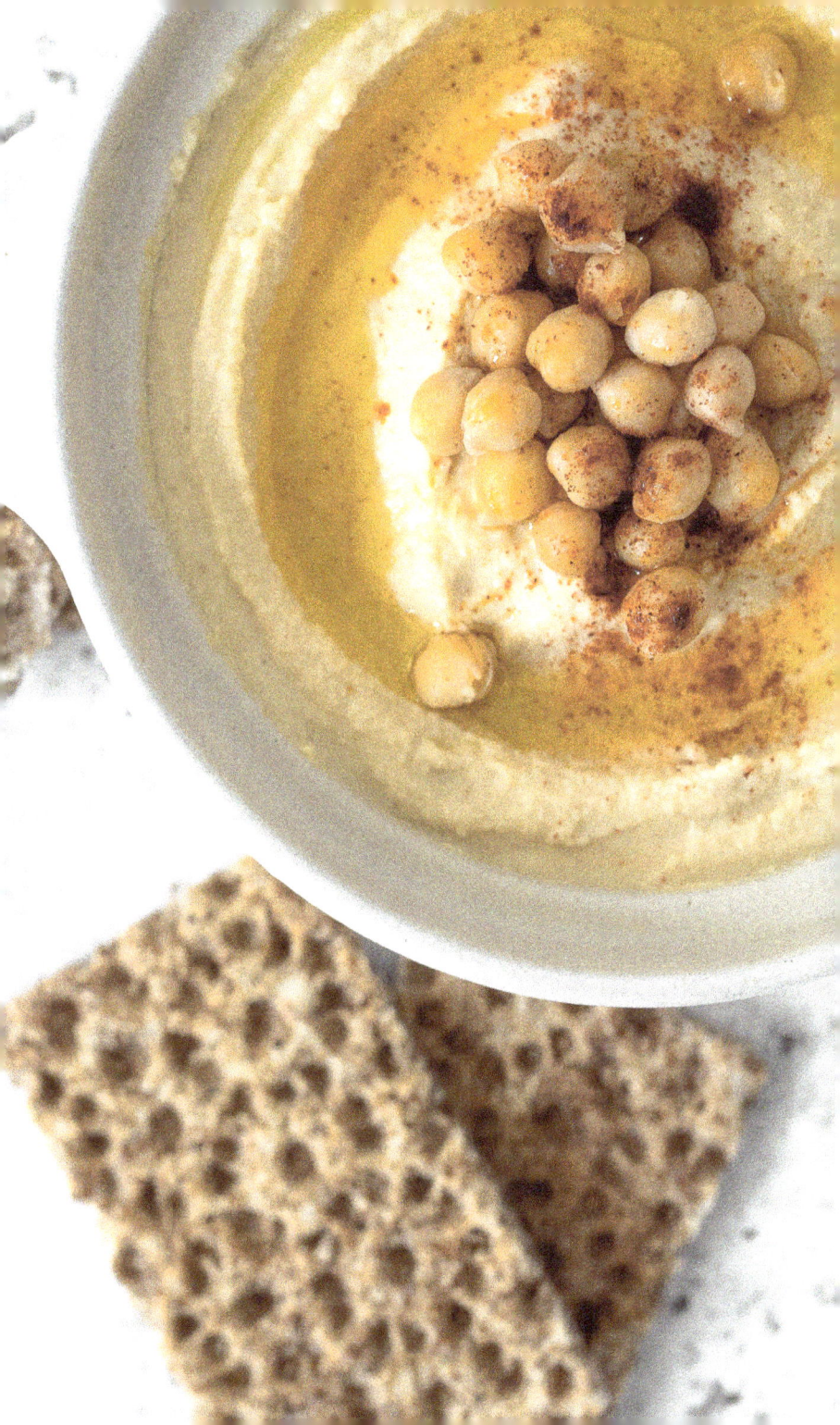

Hummus with Crackers

2 cups boiled chickpeas

1 ½ cups chickpea stock (or water if using cans)

1 tbsp tahini paste

1 pitta bread

¾ cup sugar free yoghurt (almond or soy)

2 garlic cloves

Handful roasted pine nuts

1 tsp sea salt

½ tsp cumin powder

2 tbsp lemon juice

2-3 tbsp olive oil (dressing)

Sumac and red chili powder (seasoning)

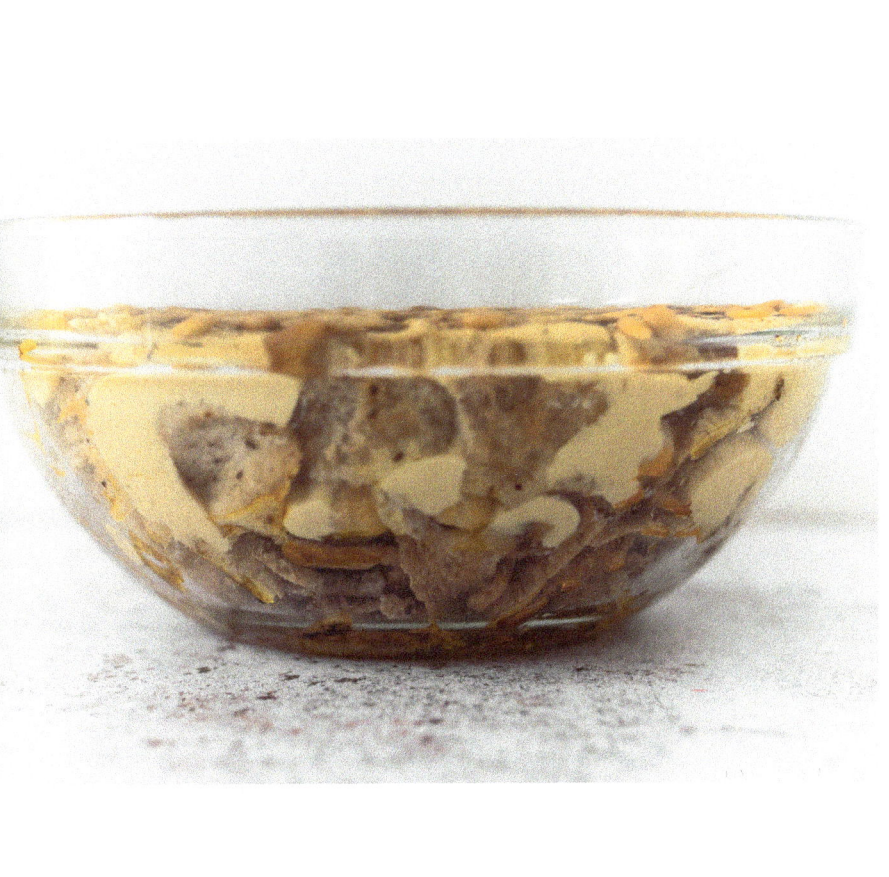

Preparation and Method

Put the pitta bread into a low heated oven (140°C) until the bread becomes dry and snappable. Snap the bread into roughly bite sized crackers and leave aside for use later.

Separate ¼ cup of chickpeas and keep aside. With the rest add, tahini, yoghurt, garlic, salt, lemon juice, chickpea stock and cumin to the blender and blend into a smooth and soft paste.

Put the ¼ cup of chickpeas into a large bowl, along with the bread crackers and then add the blended mixture on top. Top with pine nuts, sprinkle of sumac, red chili powder and finally the olive oil.

Serves 2

Tip: Almond butter can be used as an alternative to tahini paste.

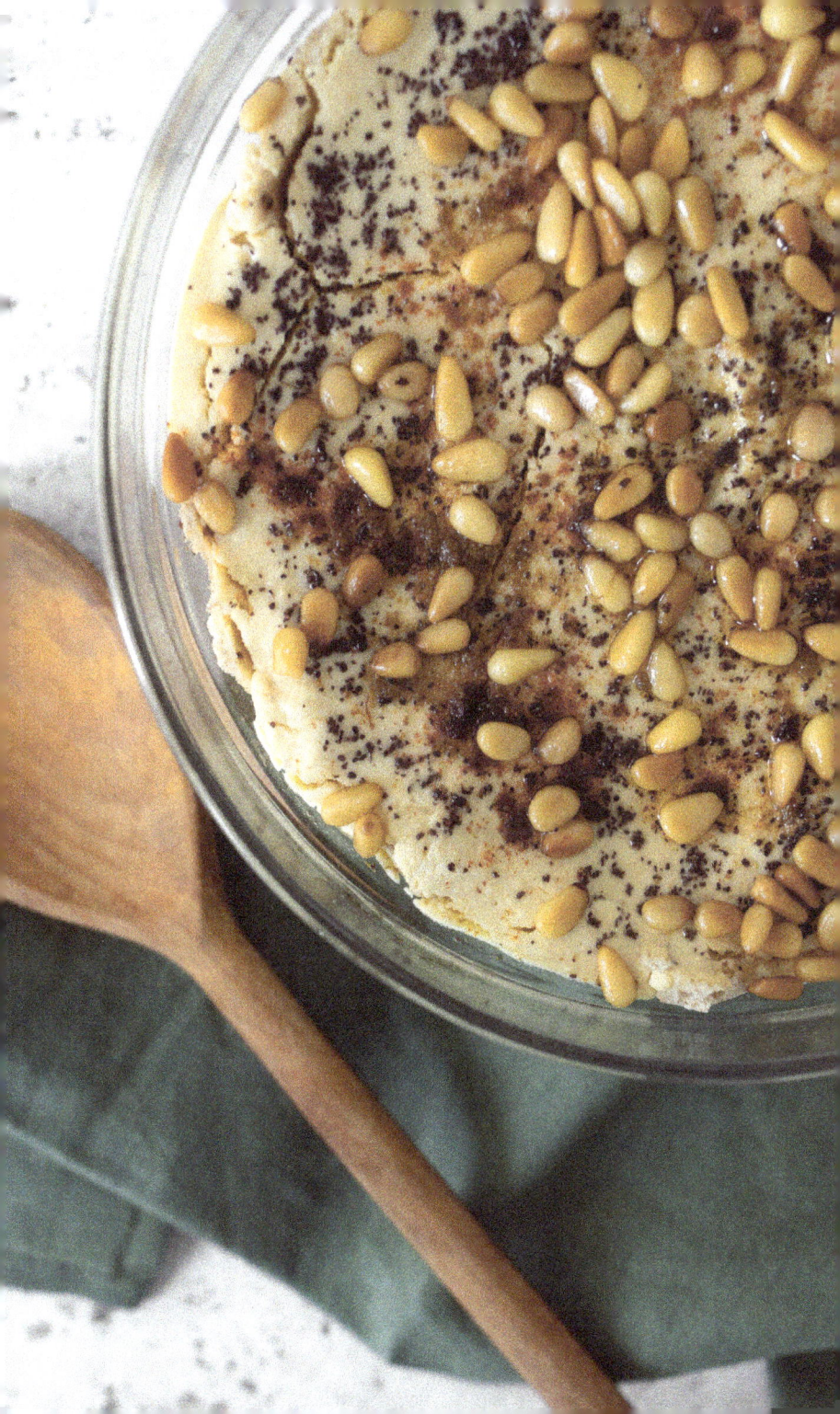

Chickpea with Aubergine

2 aubergines (egg plant)

2 cups boiled chickpeas

2 finely chopped tomatoes

2 finely chopped large onions

1 cup extra virgin olive oil

½ cup chickpea stock (or hot water if using cans)

1 ½ tbsp tomato purée

1 ½ tsp sea salt

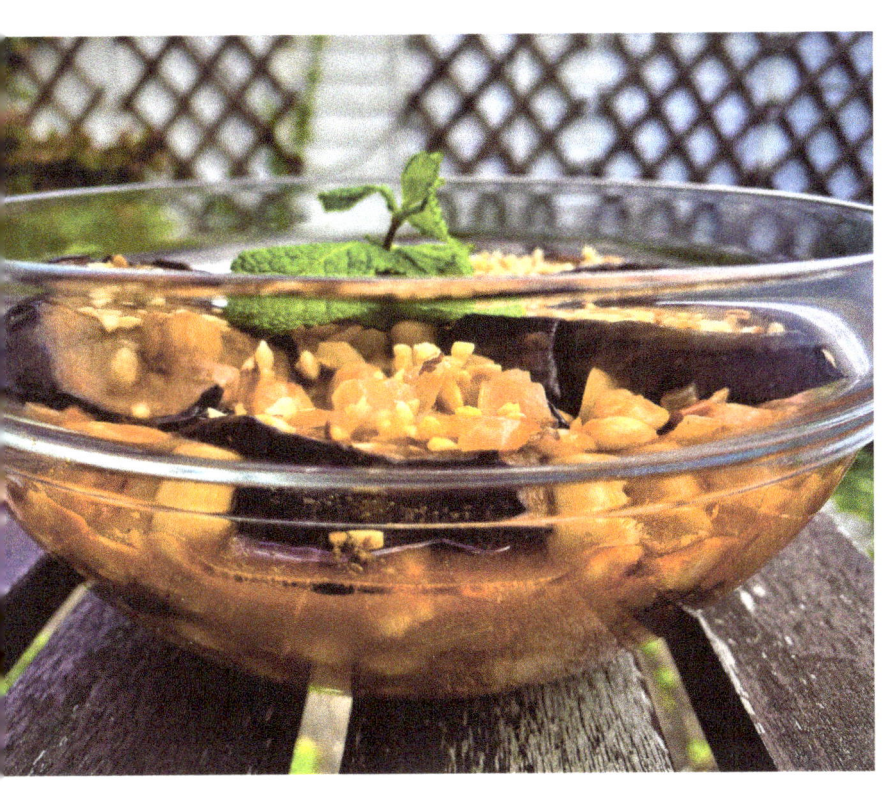

Preparation and Method

Cut the aubergines into thick slices (as pictured), brush with olive oil then grill on both sides in a preheated grill.

Sauté the chopped onions in 3 tbsp of olive oil with the chopped tomatoes and salt for 2 minutes in a saucepan. Add the tomato purée with chickpea stock into the saucepan and stir well. Then add the grilled aubergine slices. Finally, add the chickpeas with the remaining olive oil. Cover the saucepan with a lid. Wait until the mixture starts to boil then reduce the heat and leave to simmer for 30-40 minutes.

Serves 4

Tips: You can sprinkle chopped parsley, roasted pine nuts and almond flakes on top of the dish.

If you do not like tomato purée in general or avoid eating due to a health reasons such as heartburn, you can use 4 chopped tomatoes instead, omitting the use of chickpea stock or water.

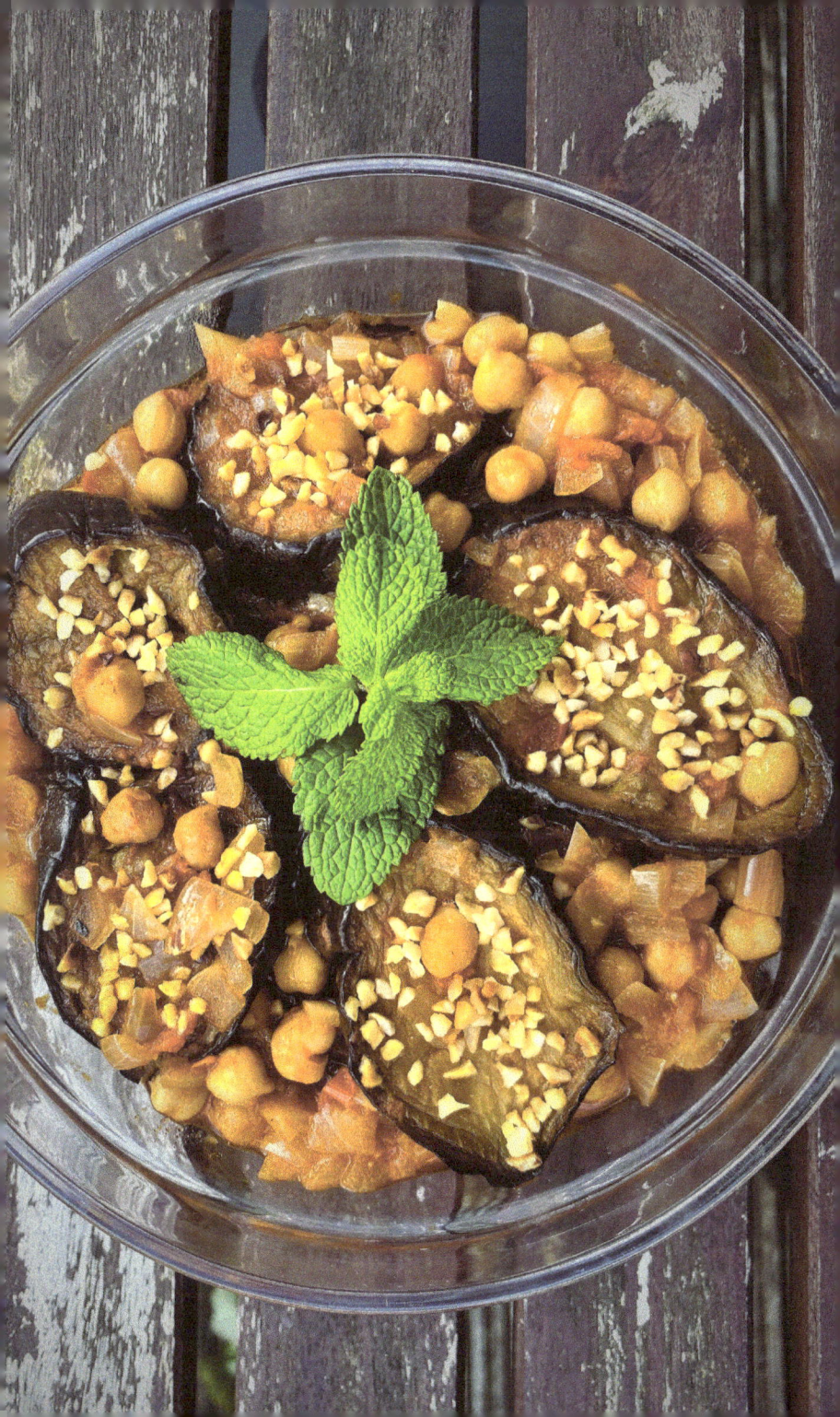

Baked Cauliflower & Chickpea with Tahini & Peanut Butter Sauce

2 small whole cauliflowers

2 cups boiled chickpeas

4 tbsp olive oil

Handful chopped parsley (topping)

3 tbsp tahini paste

2 tbsp peanut butter (no added sugar)

Juice of 2 limes

2 ½ tsp sea salt

½ tsp black pepper

4 garlic cloves

3 cups boiled water

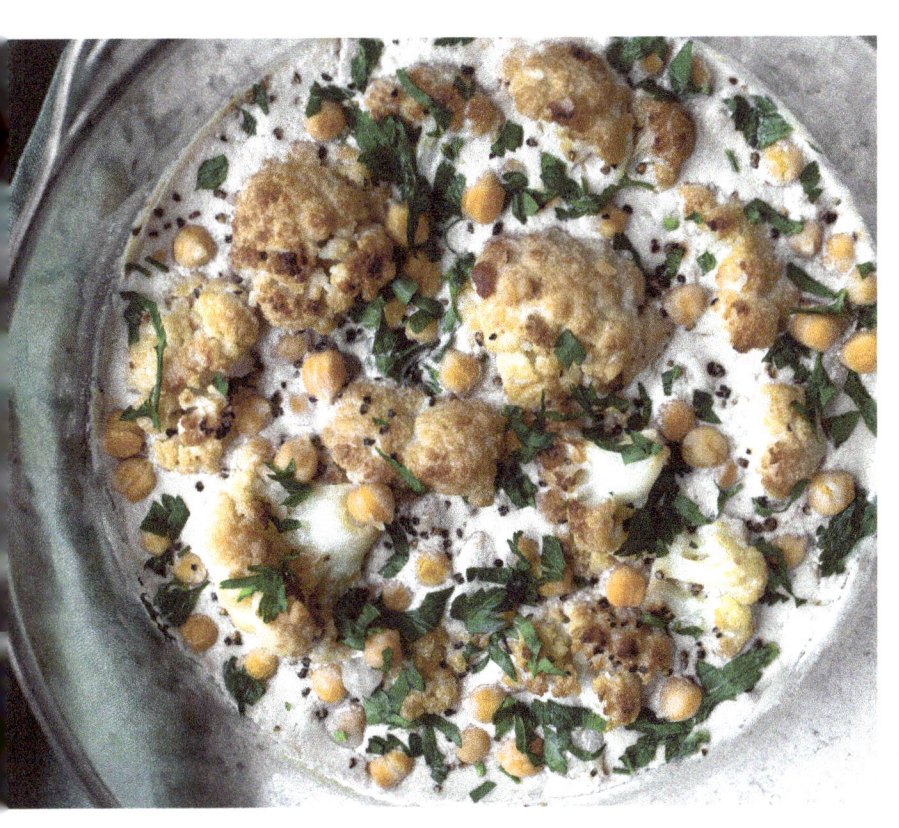

Preparation and Method

Cut the cauliflower into small chunks and place on an oven tray. Add the olive oil and rub onto the cauliflower. Grill both sides of the Cauliflower.

Put the tahini paste, peanut butter, lime juice, sea salt, black pepper, garlic cloves and boiled water into a blender and blend until smooth. This will make your sauce.

Place the grilled cauliflower onto a medium sized oven tray. Add the chickpeas, then add the sauce. Cover the tray with foil and place in a pre-heated oven at 180°C. Cook for about 25 minutes and leave to rest for 5 minutes afterwards. Sprinkle chopped parsley on top.

Serves 4-5

Tip: Delicious to be served with boiled rice or mashed potatoes.

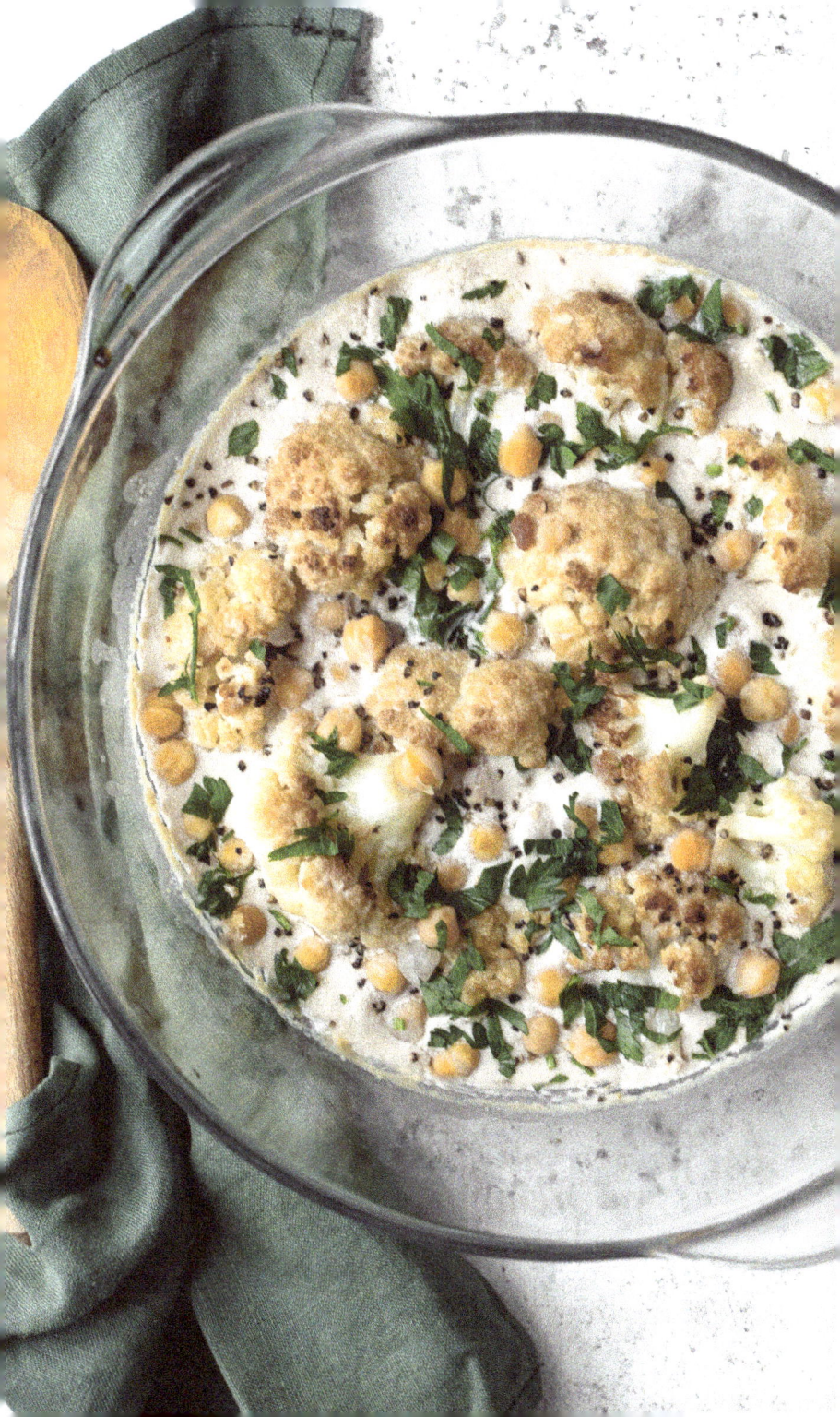

Chickpea with Bulgur

3 ½ chopped small tomatoes

1 tbsp tomato purée

1 cup chickpea stock (or hot water if using cans).

2 cups boiled chickpeas

1 cup coarse bulgur

2 chopped medium red onions

5 tbsp olive oil

1 ½ tsp sea salt

½ tsp smoke paprika (optional)

Preparation and Method

Heat 3 tbsp of olive oil in a saucepan. Add the onion and sauté for a couple of minutes. Then add the tomatoes and salt and sauté until softened. Add the tomato puree to the tomatoes and keep mixing until a paste is formed. Next add the coarse bulgur, boiled chickpeas, chickpea stock (or water) and paprika to the saucepan. Once boiling, reduce the heat and leave to simmer for 30 minutes.

Switch off the heat and leave to rest for 5 minutes before serving.

Serves 3

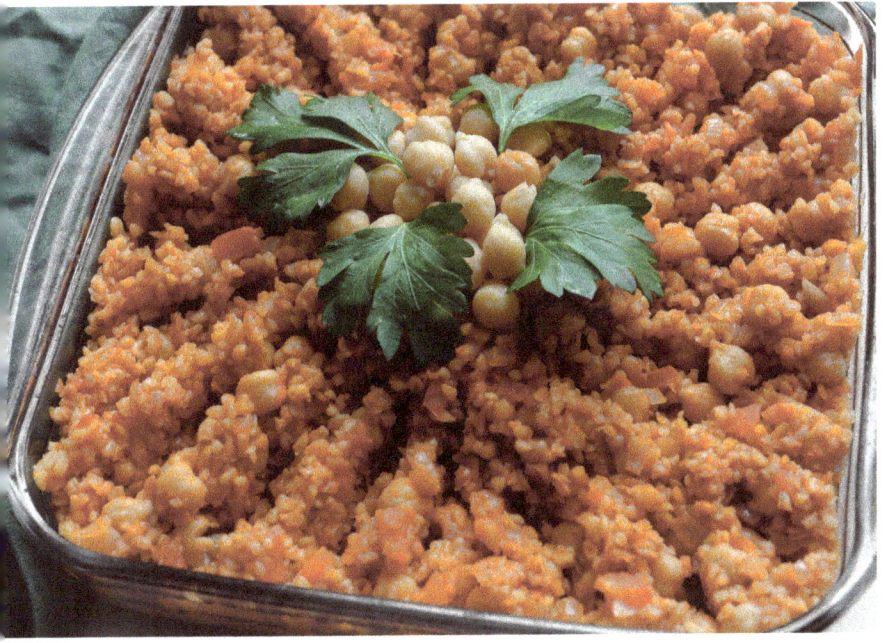

Fava/Broad Beans

- Fava beans are very high in protein and have the ability to make you feel full for a long time.

- They are popular in Egypt and the wider Levantine area.

- Dry fava beans are treated the same as other dry beans before cooking i.e., washed and soaked in water for about 24 hours whilst refreshing the water twice within that time frame before cooking. However hot water is used instead of cold.

- The initial cooking time is longer than other beans, approximately 4 hours. To reduce the cooking time, add ¼ - ½ tsp of bicarbonate of soda (note: bicarbonate of soda can mildly influence the taste).

- To save energy, money and time, soak and cook a large quantity of fava beans, then divide into smaller portions and store in the freezer. They can then be used later to quickly prepare the delicious meals explained in the following pages.

- There are two kinds of fava beans, large and small. I personally prefer the smaller ones as I find them to be tastier in meals. One of my favorite meals is the 'Fava Bean and Chickpea Dip'. I am also a fan of skinless fava beans as they tend to have a softer texture and take less time to cook.

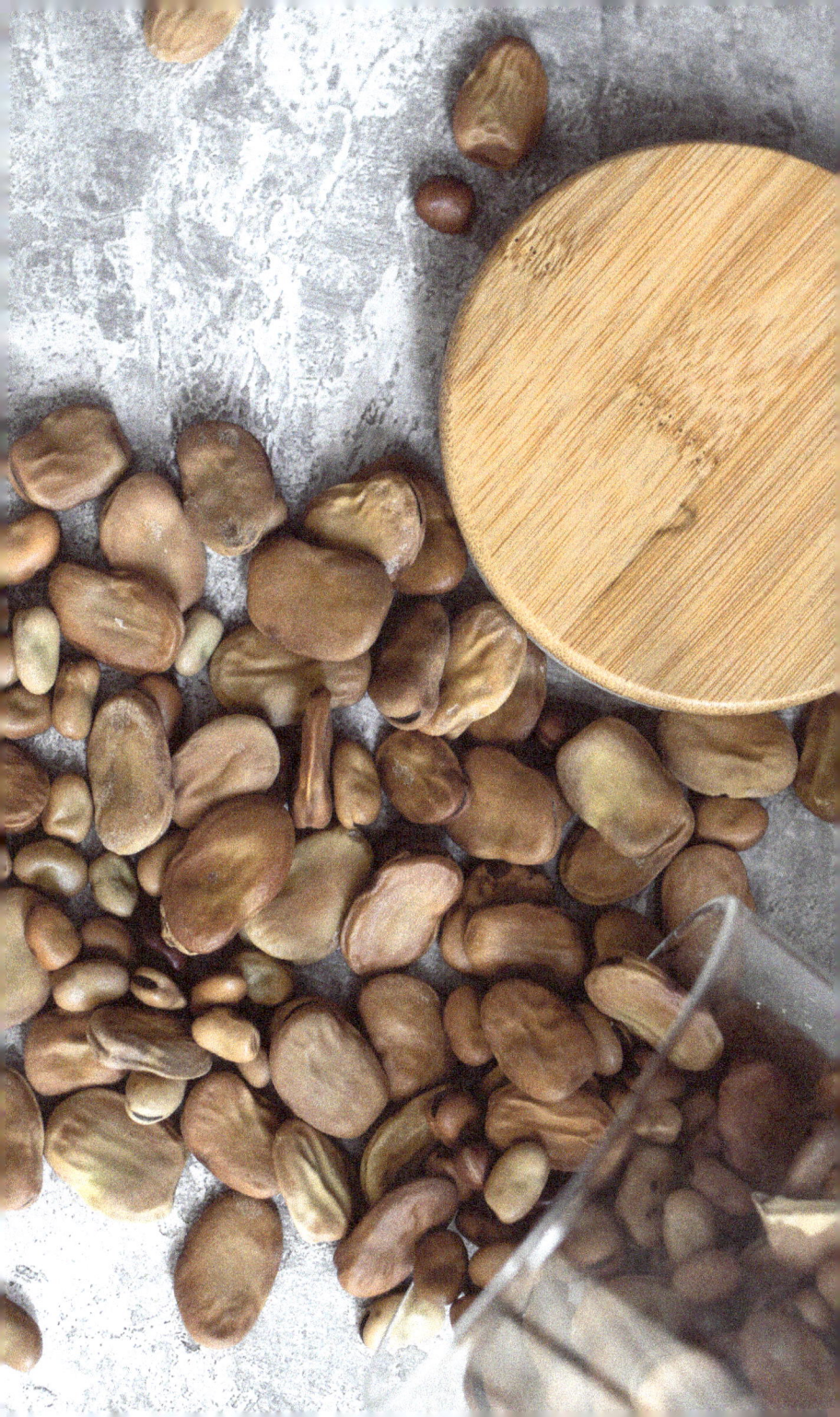

Fava Bean & Chickpea Dip

3 cups boiled fava beans

2 cups boiled chickpeas

1 finely chopped onion

1 finely chopped tomato

½ cup boiled water

Juice of 1 lime/lemon

2 tsp sea salt

1 ½ tsp cumin powder

5 crushed garlic cloves

1 heaped tbsp tahini paste

3 tbsp extra virgin olive oil

2 tbsp extra virgin olive oil (dressing)

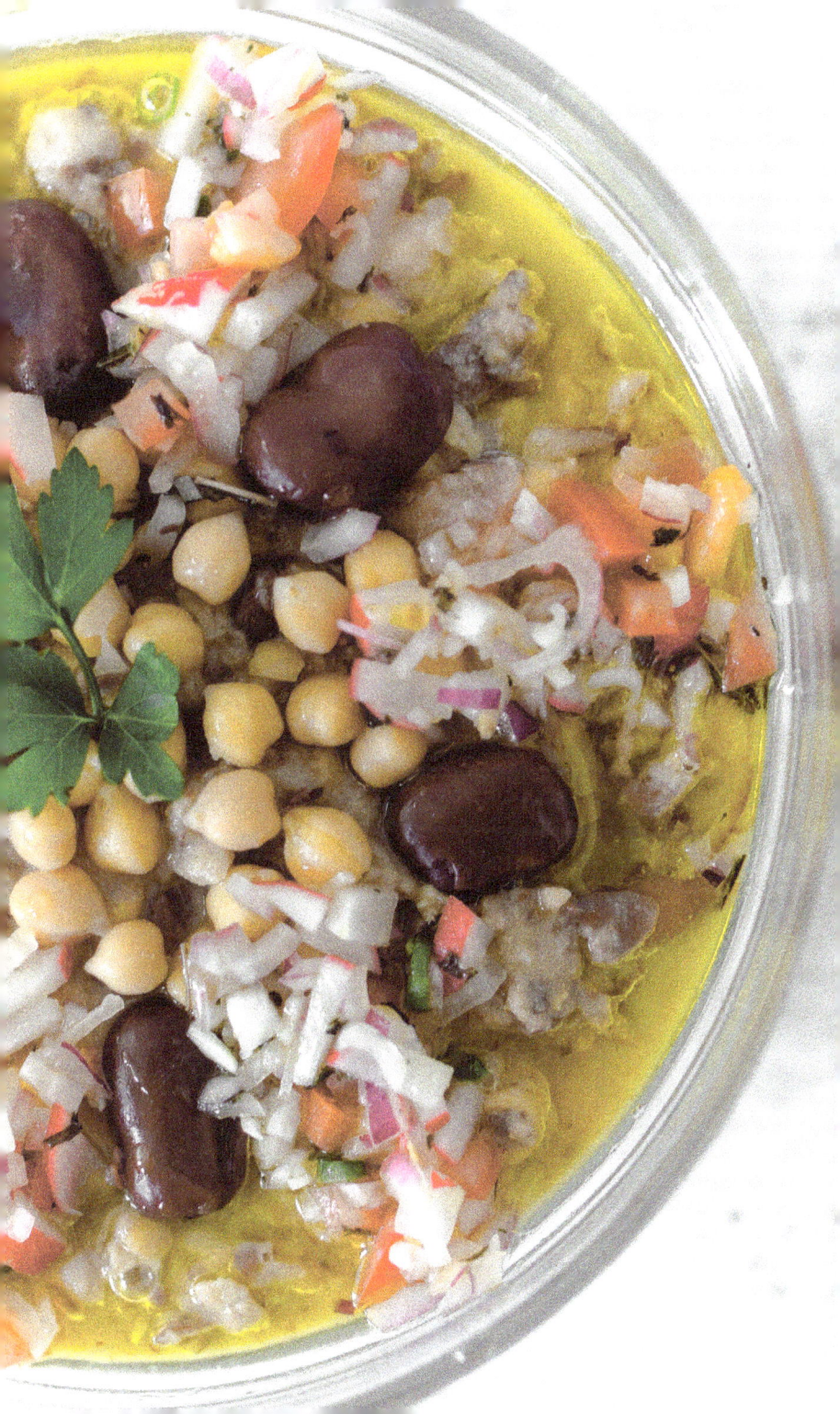

Preparation and Method

Mash the fava beans and chickpeas with a potato masher in a saucepan. Add all the other ingredients. Bring the mixture to boil then reduce the heat and leave to simmer for 15 minutes.

Tips: You can make a variation of this recipe using 5 cups of fava beans and no chickpeas. Additionally, applying a generous topping of extra virgin olive oil will provide extra flavour.

For people who tend to feel bloated after eating pulses, you can add ½ tsp of aniseed powder to the mixture whilst it is cooking to reduce bloating effects. Serves 4

Note: When reheating, add a little water to reduce the thickness.

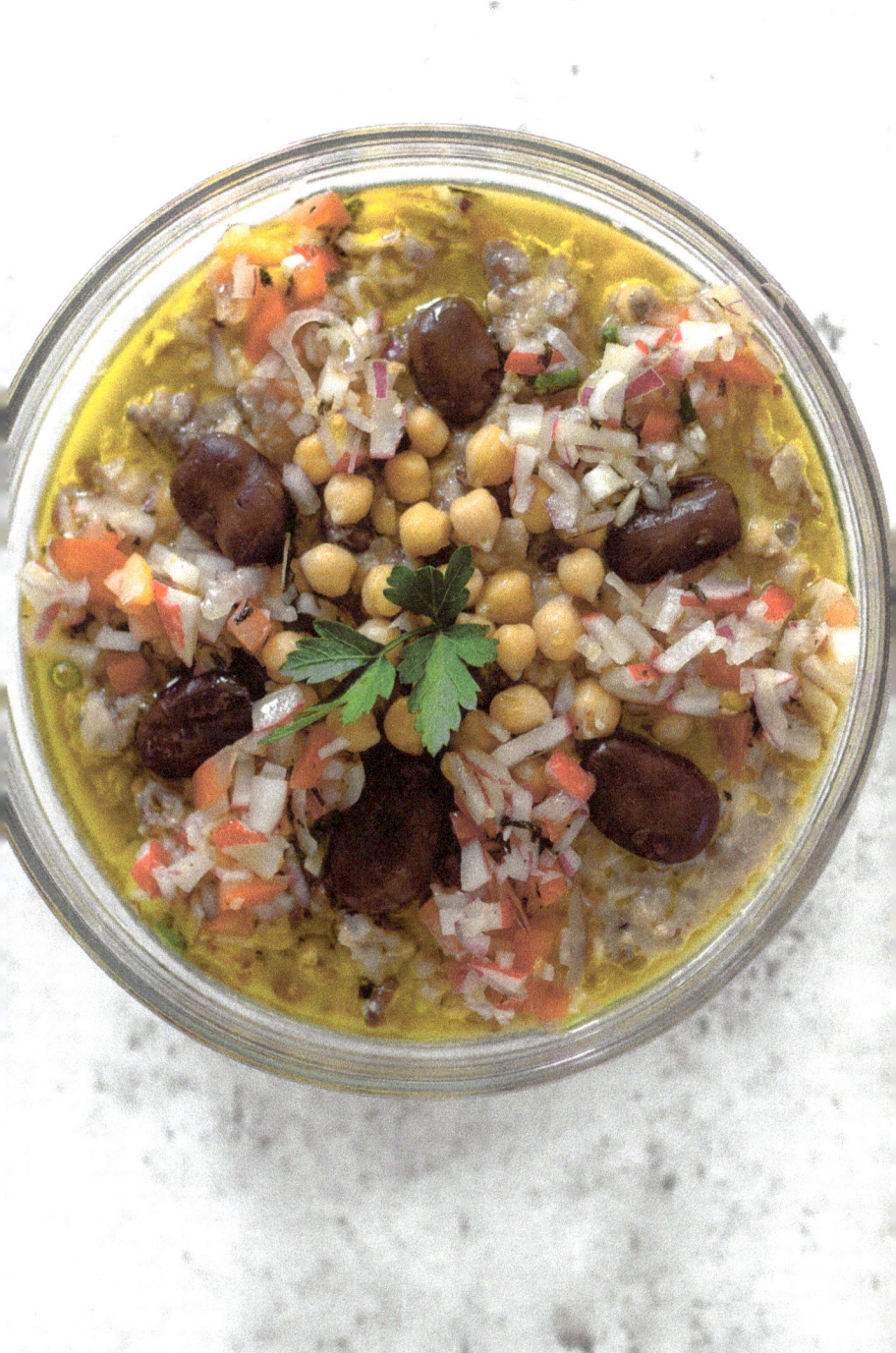

Skinless Fava Bean with Dry Mallow Dip

1 cup dried skinless fava beans

2 ½ cups water

1 cup dry mallow leaves

1 crushed garlic head

5 tbsp olive oil

½ lemon juice

½ tsp red chili flakes

1 tsp salt

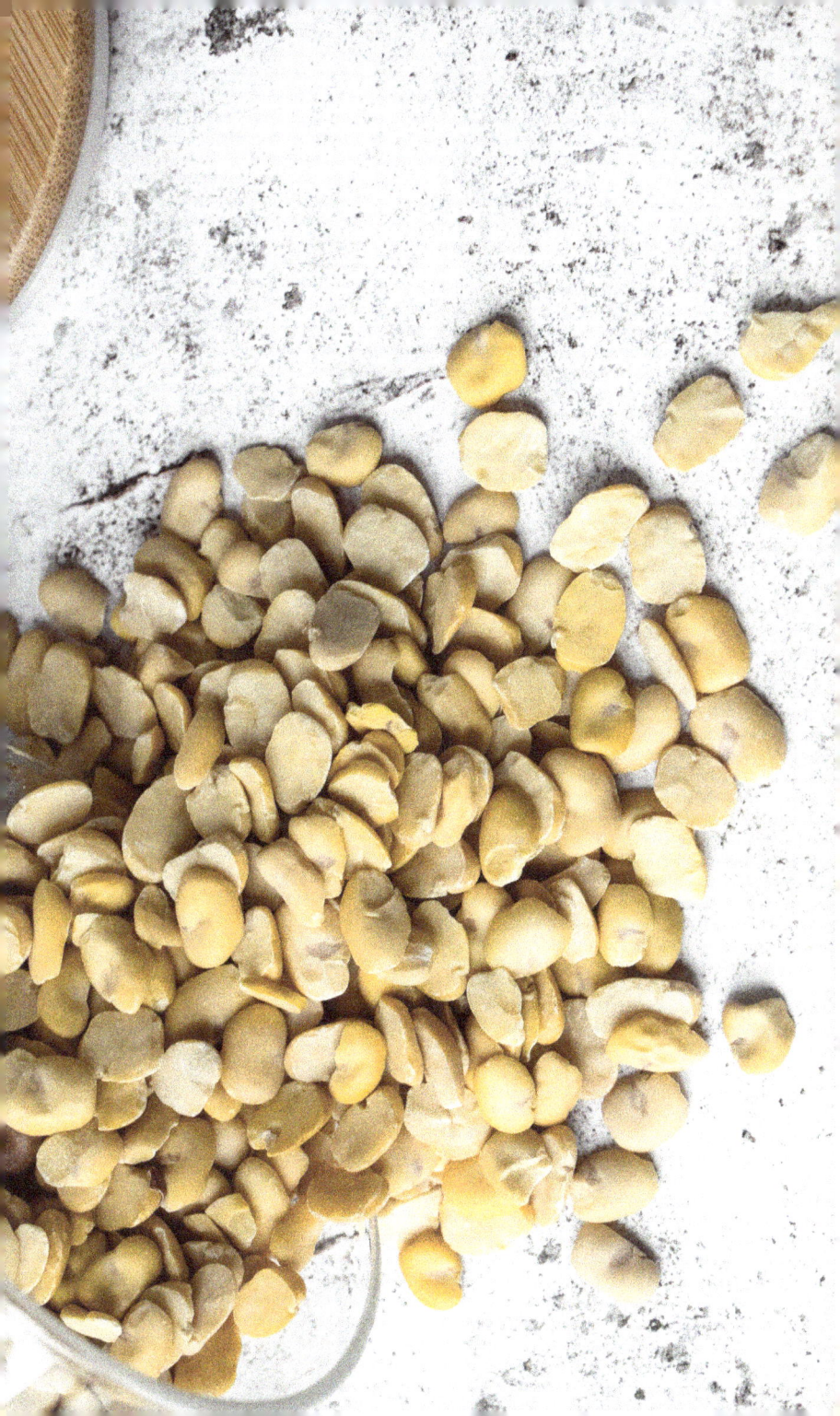

Preparation and Method

Wash the fava beans and add them to a saucepan with the water. Bring to boil then reduce the heat to allow it to simmer. When you first reduce the heat, collect and remove the foam that forms on top of the water, without removing any water. After 30 minutes, add the dry mallow. Leave to simmer for a further 25-30 minutes.

Whilst the beans cook, sauté the garlic with 3 tbsp of olive oil until softened. 10 minutes before switching off the heat, add the garlic, salt, lemon juice, red chili and 2 tbsp of olive oil to the beans. You can eat it hot or cold.

Serve with pitta bread, breadsticks or spread it on toast.

Serves 2

Note: Instead of dry mallow, you can use 2 cups of freshly chopped spinach.

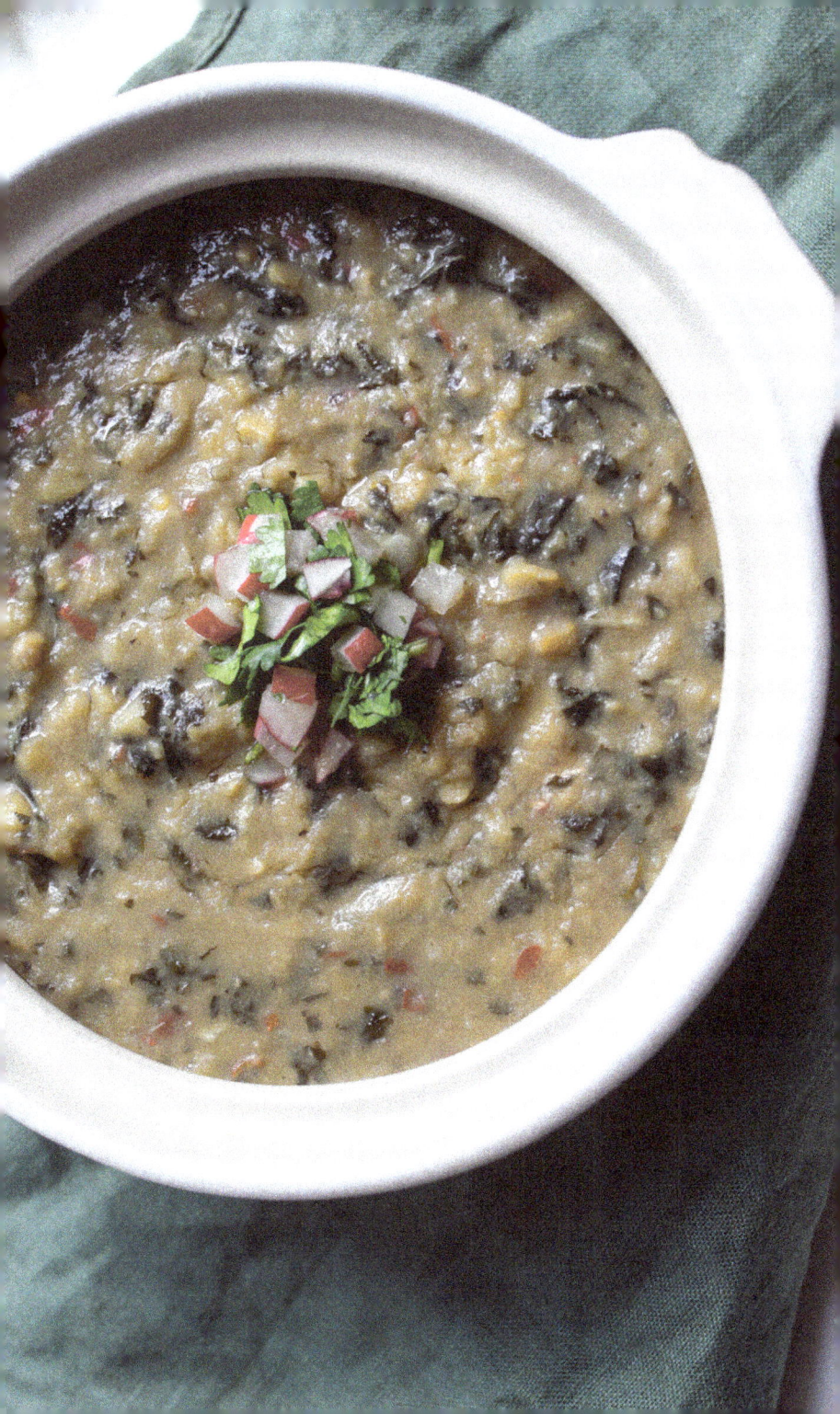

Skinless Fava Bean with Peanut Butter Pâte

1 cup dried skinless fava beans

2 ½ cups water

1 tsp sea salt

1 crushed garlic clove

2 tbsp olive oil

1 tbsp lime juice

3 tbsp peanut butter (no added sugar)

½ tsp harissa paste (optional)

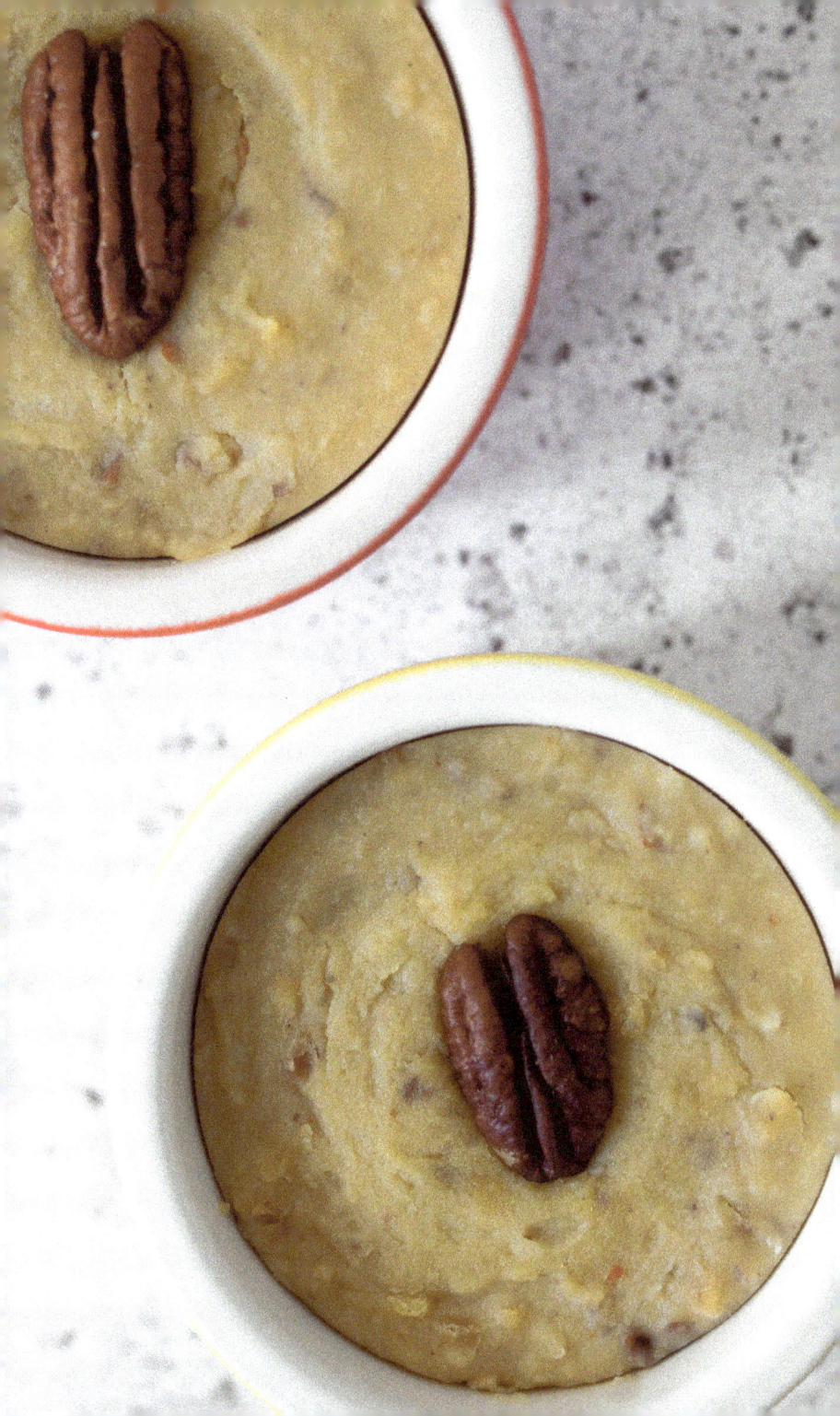

Preparation and Method

Wash the beans with fresh water. Put in a saucepan with 2½ cups of water and bring to boil, then turn the heat down and leave to simmer for about 50 minutes. Whilst the beans cook, sauté the garlic with 2 tbsp of olive oil. Then add to the beans in the saucepan, along with the salt.

Once done, pour the mixture into a blender and add the peanut butter, lime juice and harissa. Then blend until smooth. Return the mixture to the saucepan and over a medium heat, stir for another 5 minutes.

Empty the mixture into a small bowl and leave to cool. It is best served cold.

Serves 2

Note: If you like your peanut butter crunchy, do not blend, just add to the mixture in the saucepan in the last 5 minutes.

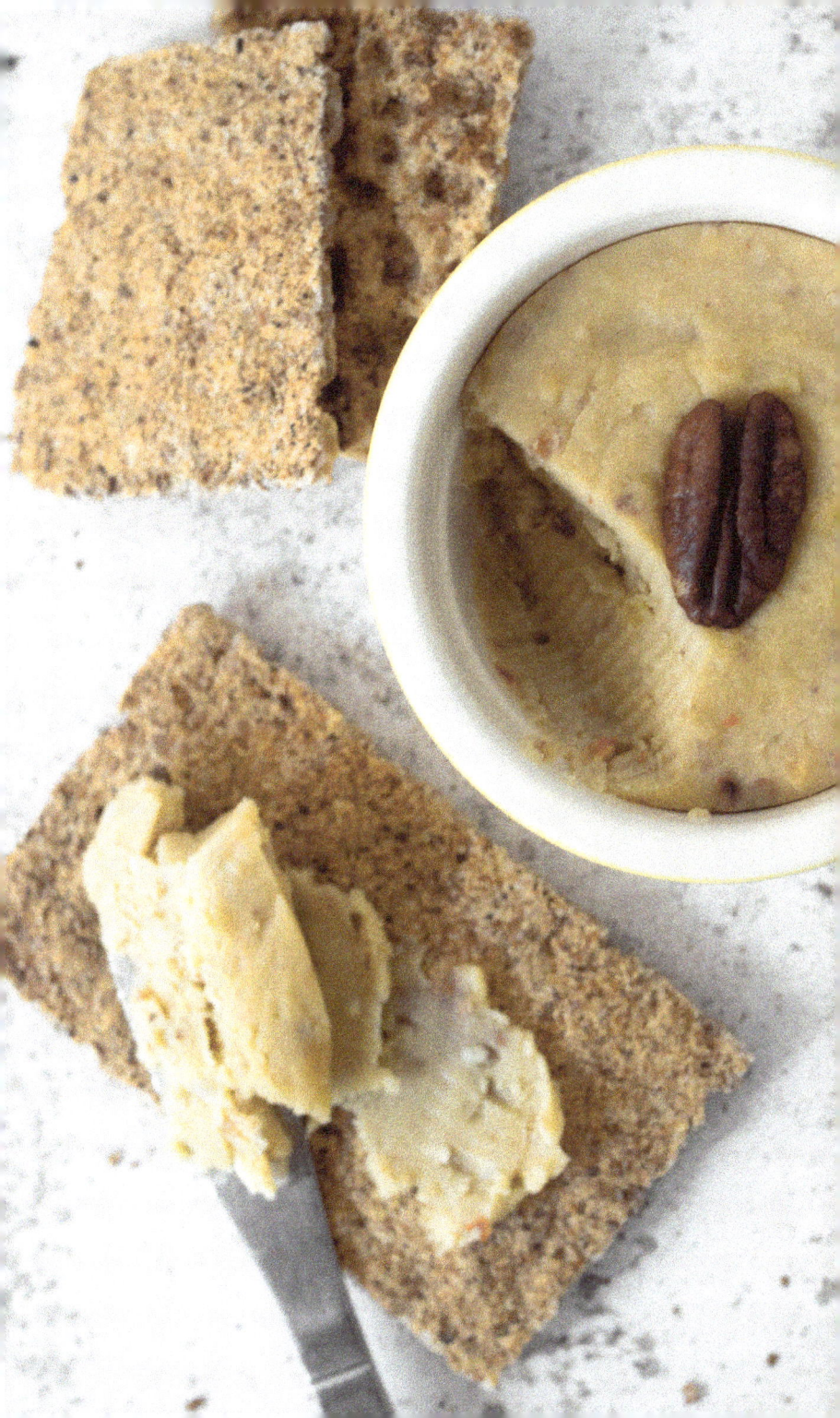

Dried Peas

Peas contain various amounts of nutrients. They are a very good source of potassium, copper, manganese, pantothenic acid, phosphorus and folate. 500g of dry split peas equates to about 6 cups after being soaked in water overnight.

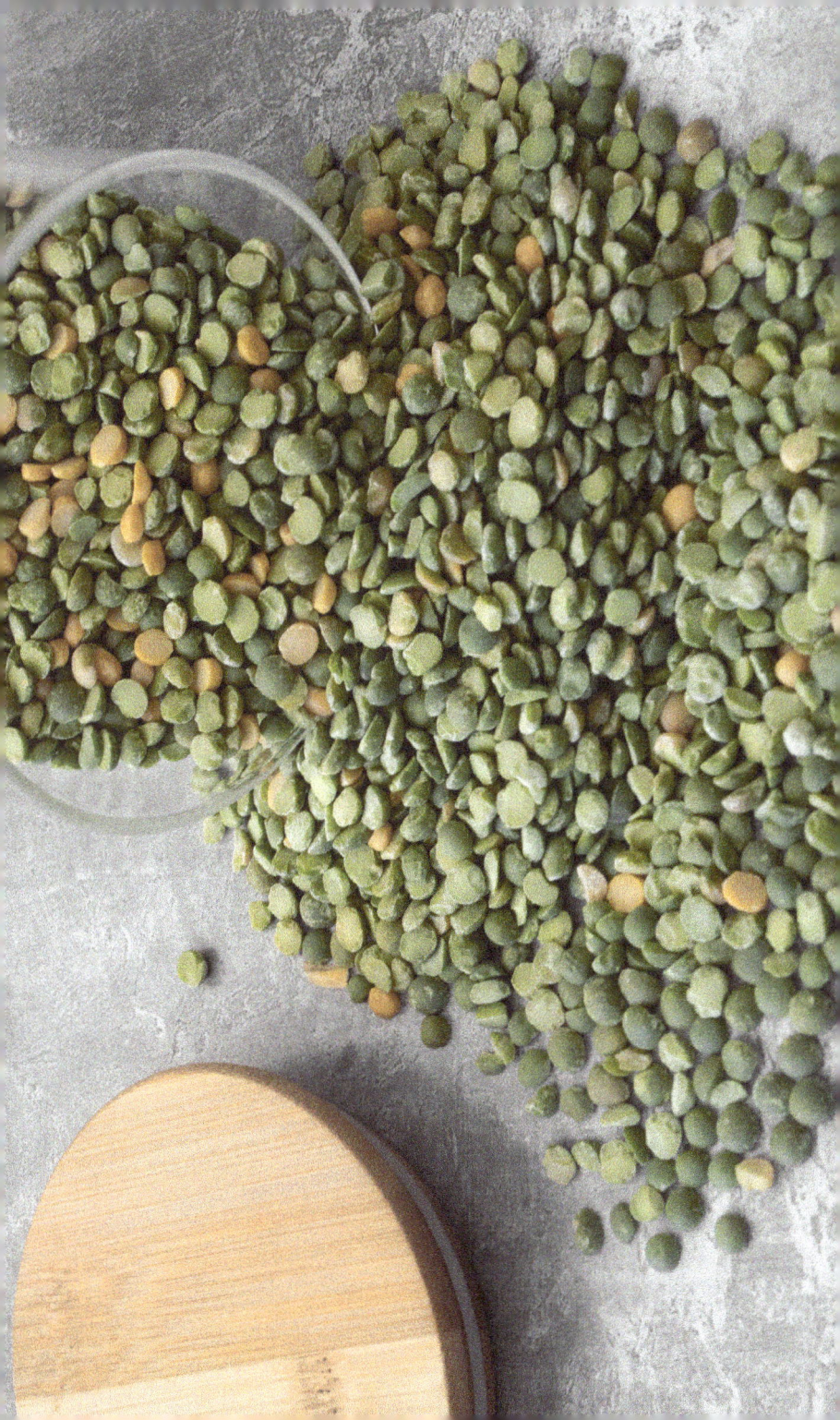

Falafel Spices

Falafel is traditionally made from either skinless fava beans or chickpeas, and sometimes a mixture of both. In my recipe, I have only used dried peas that have been soaked overnight which I have found to be a very tasty alternative to traditional falafels. The following falafel recipe's main spices can be found in the form of seeds which you can grind before using or as a powder. Alternatively, you can buy falafel spices ready made from middle eastern food stores.

1 tbsp cumin

1 tbsp coriander

1 tsp black pepper

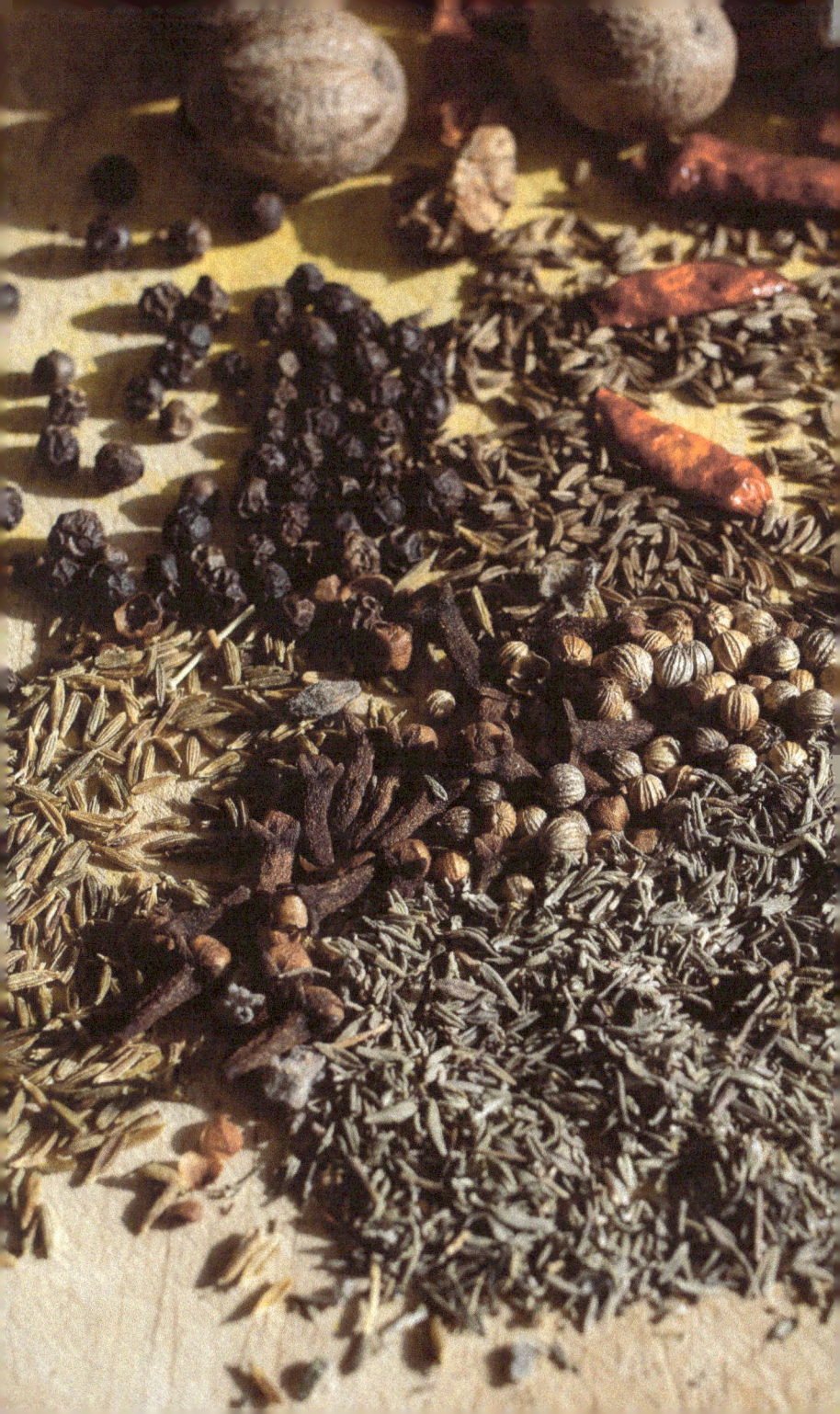

Baked or Fried Pea Falafel with Tahini Sauce

1 cup dried peas soaked in water overnight

3 garlic cloves

1 small onion

1 tsp sea salt

1 ½ tsp falafel spices

1 tsp baking powder

2 tbsp chopped coriander

2 tbsp chopped dill

1 ½ tbsp water

2 ½ cups cooking oil (if frying)

3-5 tbsp olive oil (if baking)

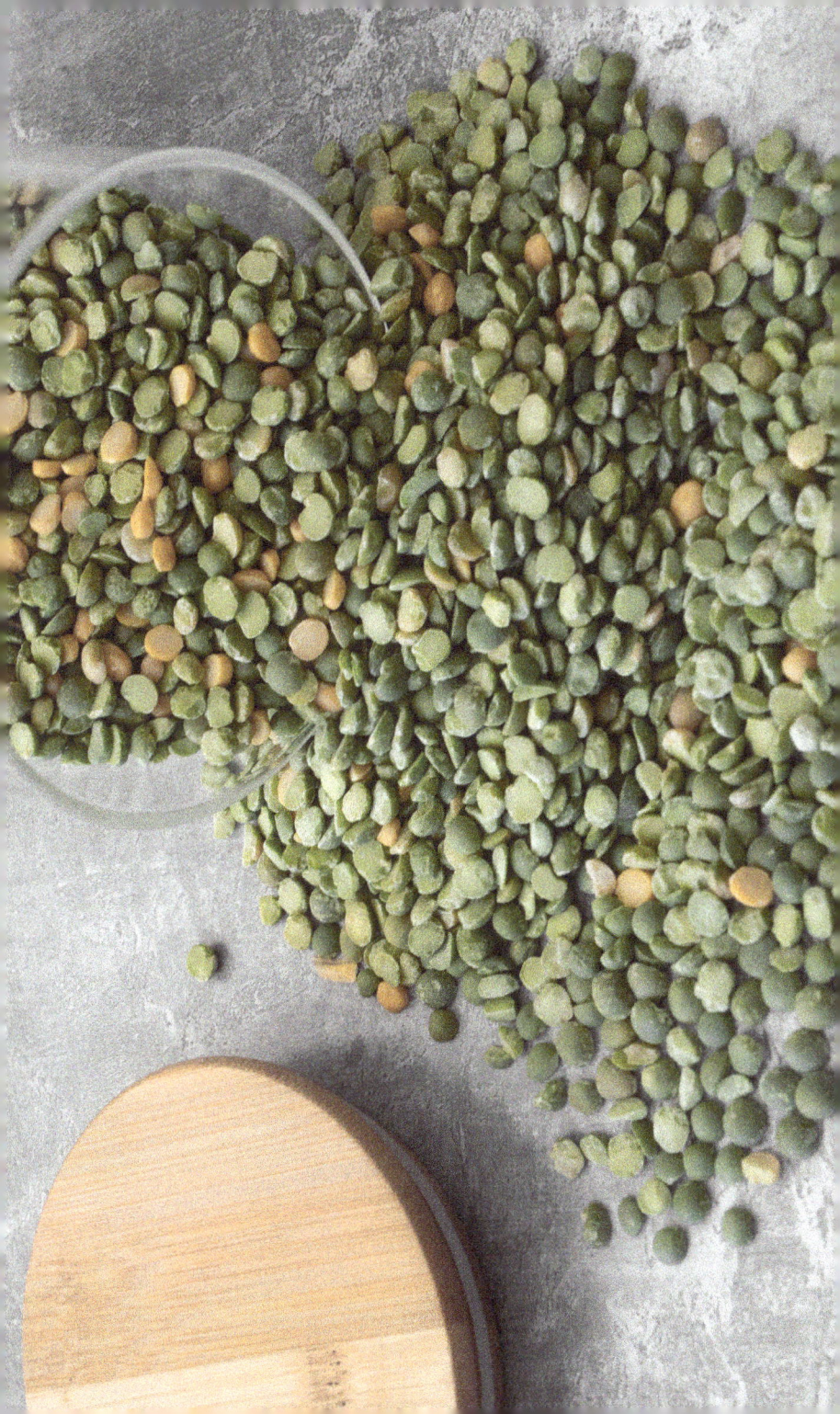

Preparation and Method

Wash the soaked peas and place them in a blender with the salt, garlic, onion, spices, coriander, dill, olive oil and 1½ tbsp of water.

Once the mixture is smooth, remove from the blender and leave to rest for an hour in the fridge.

Mix in the baking powder by hand and divide into small or medium sized balls. Brush the baking tray with a generous amount of cooking oil or use baking parchment and place the balls in the tray. Place the tray in the middle of a 180°c preheat oven for about 20 minutes then turn the falafels upside down and bake for another 10 minutes.

For frying: Fry in hot cooking oil, turning them as they turn golden brown.

Serves 3-4

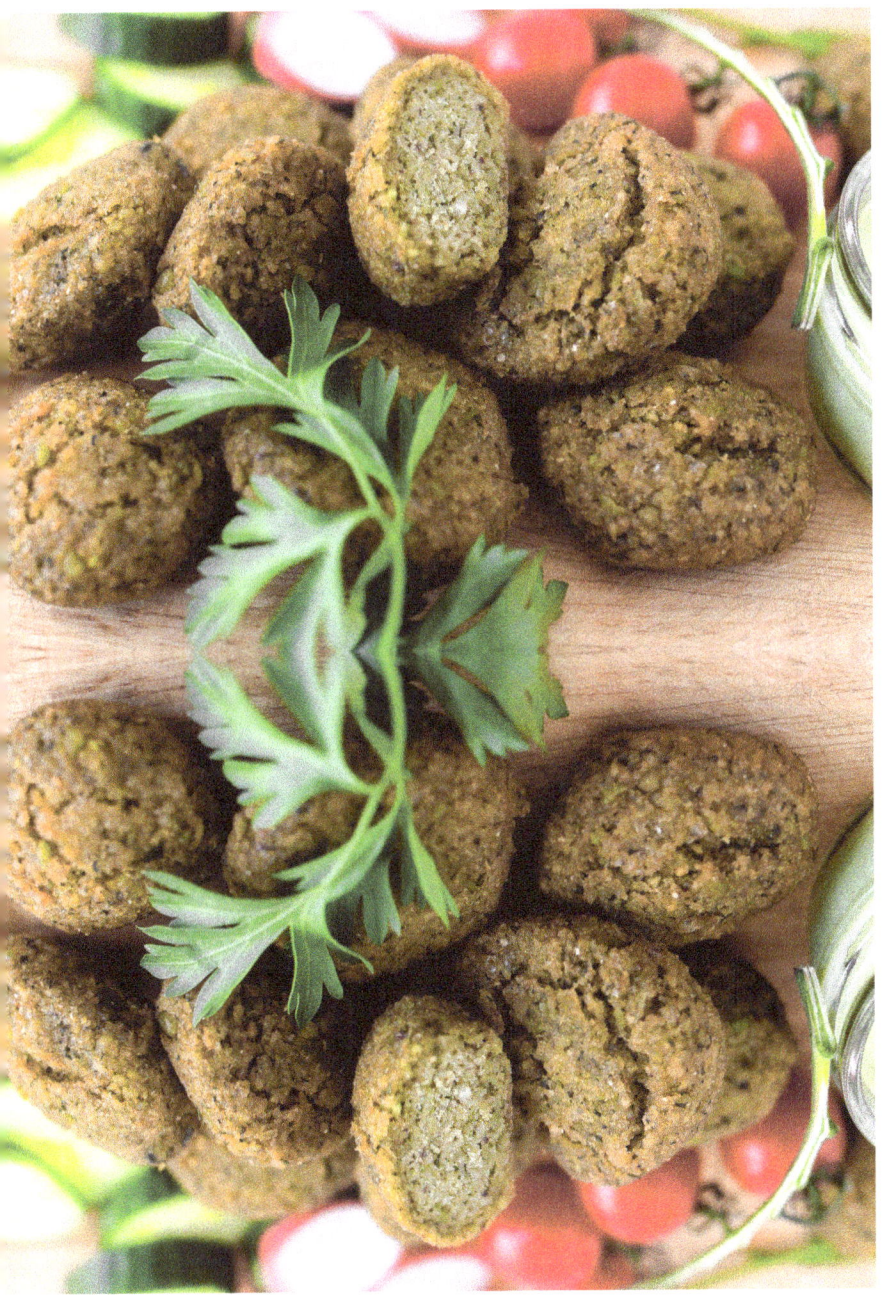

Tahini Sauce

Place into the blender:

1 garlic clove

2 tbsp lemon juice

½ tsp salt

2 tbsp tahini paste

1 cup water

Handful chopped parsley

Blend into a creamy paste.

To be served in pitta bread or wraps with slices of tomato and tahini sauce.

Tip: Peanut or almond butter can be used as an alternative to tahini paste.

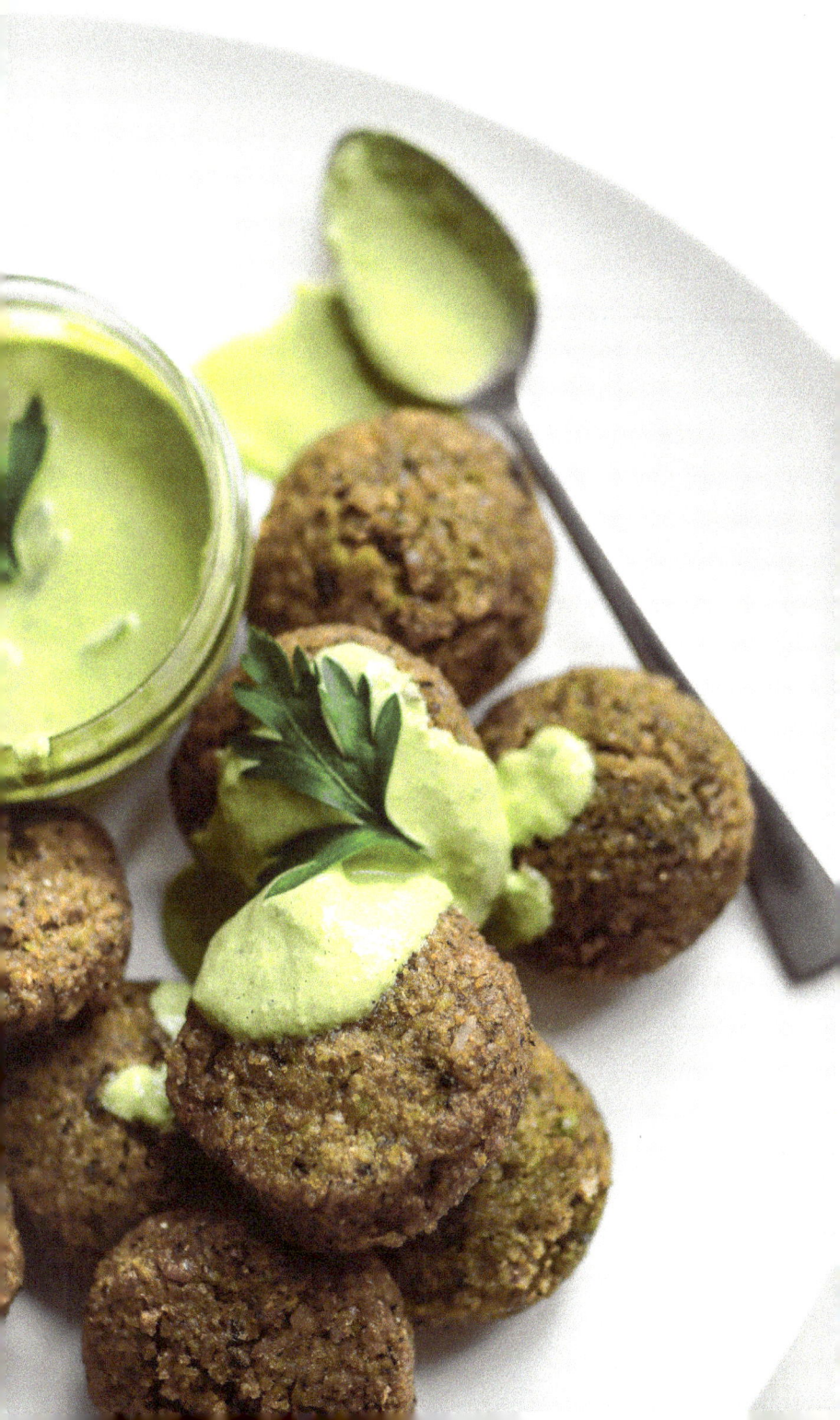

Quinoa

Quinoa originates from South America and contains all the essential amino acids that our bodies are unable to make naturally, otherwise known as being a 'complete protein.

Quinoa does not contain gluten, meaning it is suitable for people who are sensitive to gluten and additionally is rich in fibre. Quinoa comes in a variety of colours.

Cooking time 15-20 minutes.

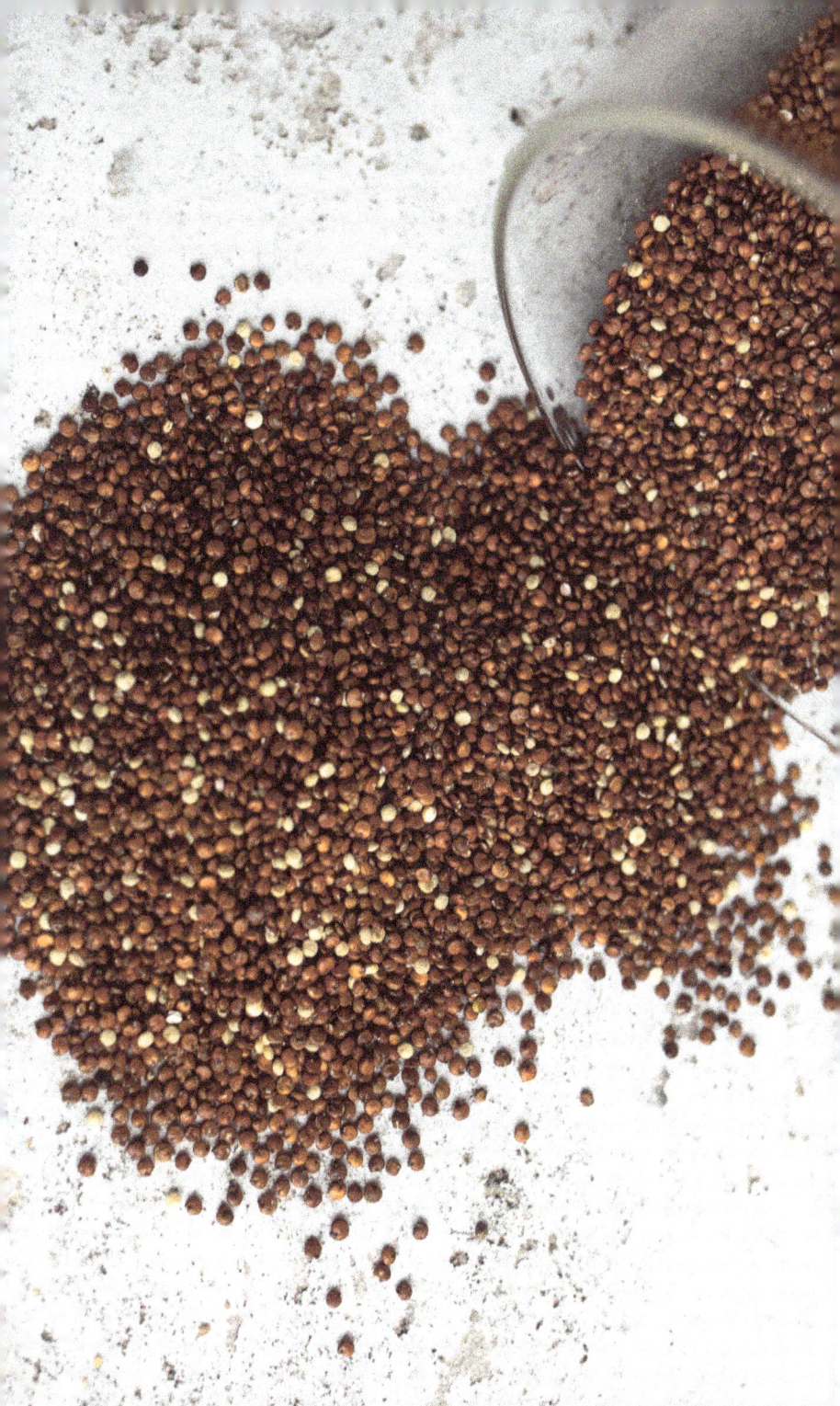

Dried Peas with Quinoa

2 cups boiled dried peas

1 ¾ cups boiled brown or white quinoa

5 tbsp olive oil

4 crushed garlic cloves

1 medium sized chopped onion

1 tbsp tomato purée

2 large chopped boiled carrots

1 ¼ tsp sea salt

½ cup chopped parsley

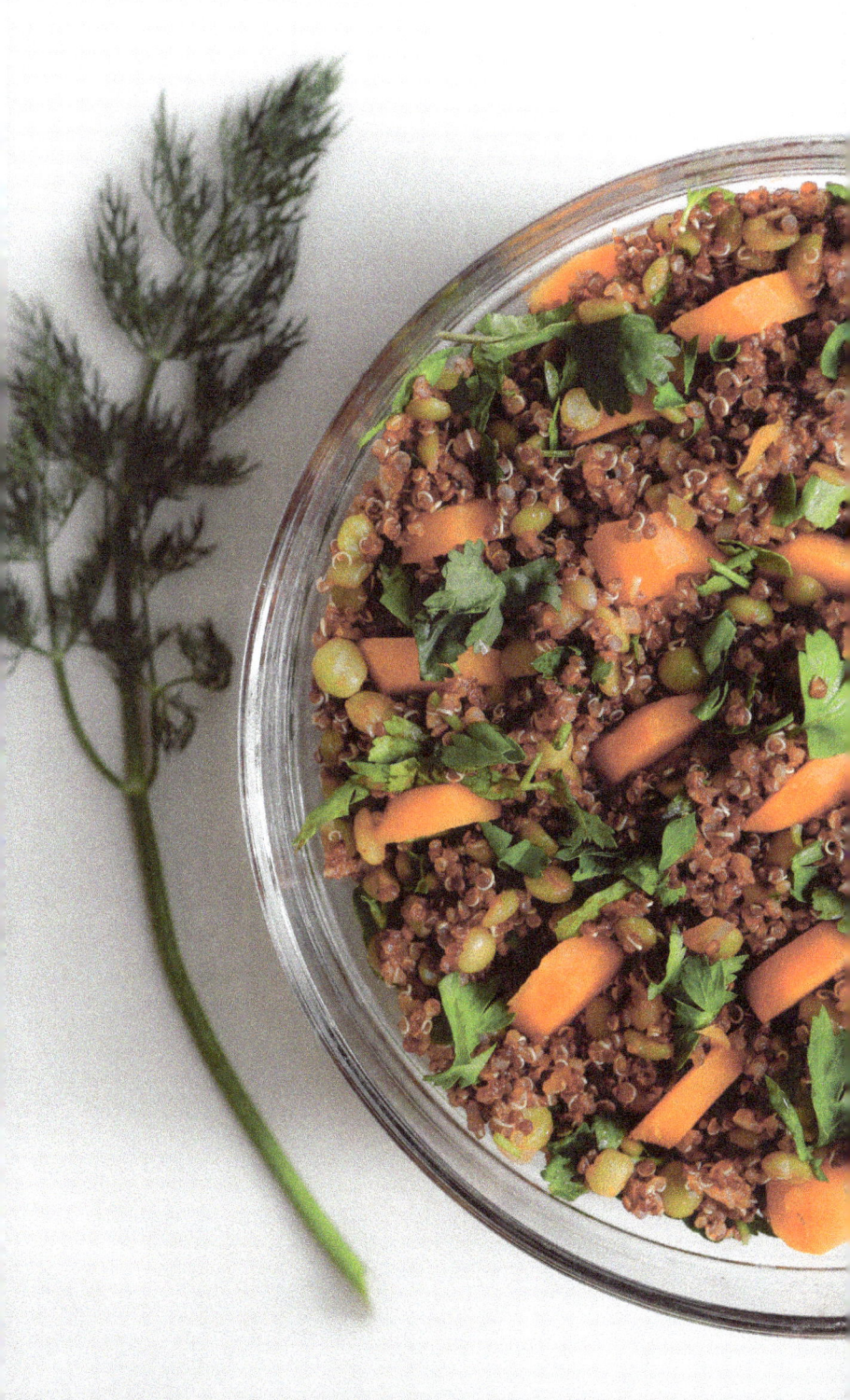

Preparation and Method

Heat 5 tbsp of olive oil in a saucepan. Add the chopped onion and crushed garlic, and sauté for a few minutes until softened. Next add the tomato puree and salt and keep stirring until a paste-like mixture is formed. Finally add the boiled dried peas, quinoa, carrots and mix together. Switch off the heat and empty mixture into a big bowl and then mix in the chopped parsley.

Serves 2

Tip: Delicious served with plain yoghurt.

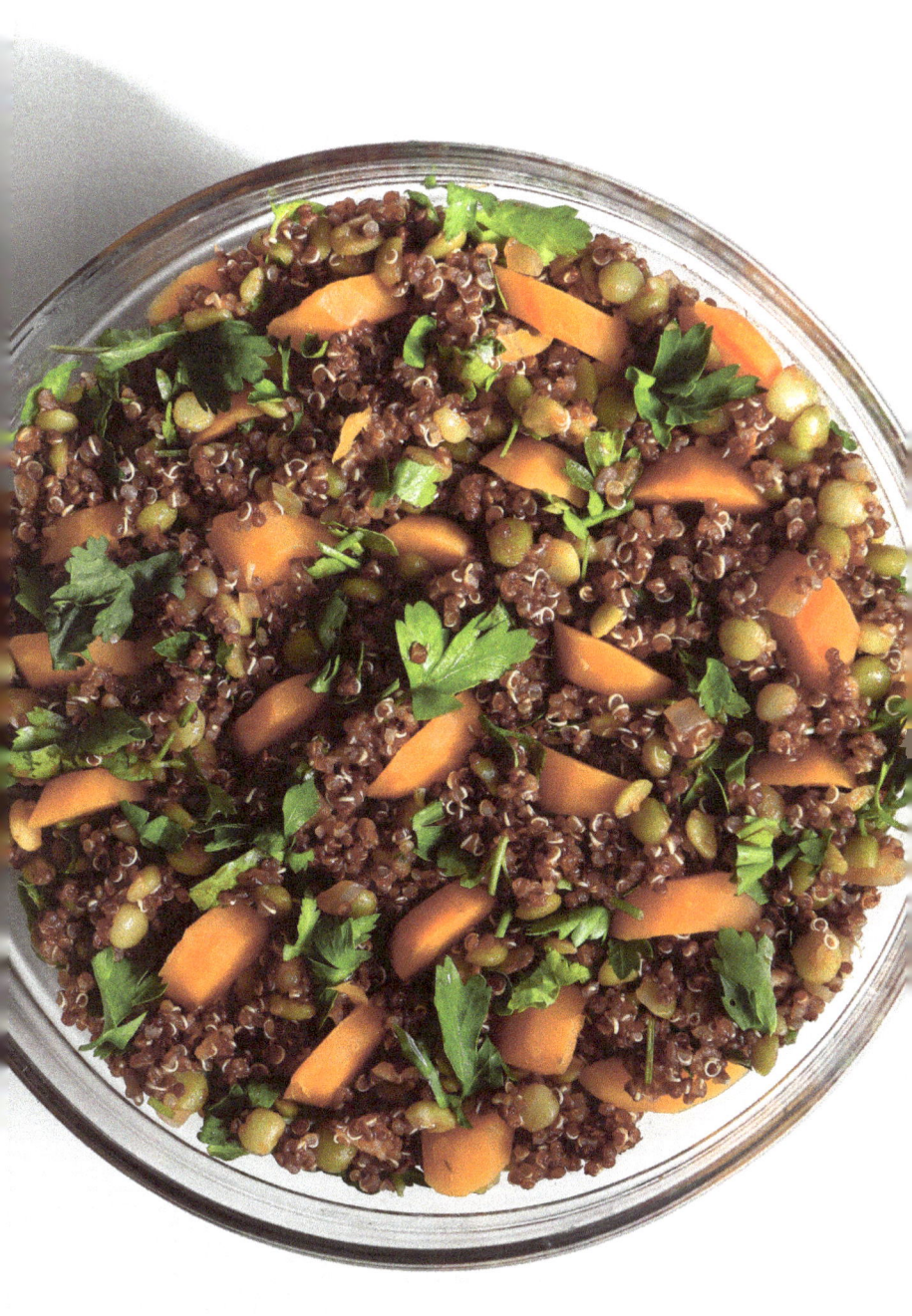

Kabsa Spices

1 tbsp dry lemon powder

5 tbsp curry powder

1 tbsp cardamom

1 tbsp cinnamon

1 tbsp turmeric

1 tbsp ginger

3 cloves

Mix the above ingredients together and store the powder in a jar, ready for use. Alternatively, you can find kabsa spices ready made in middle eastern food stores.

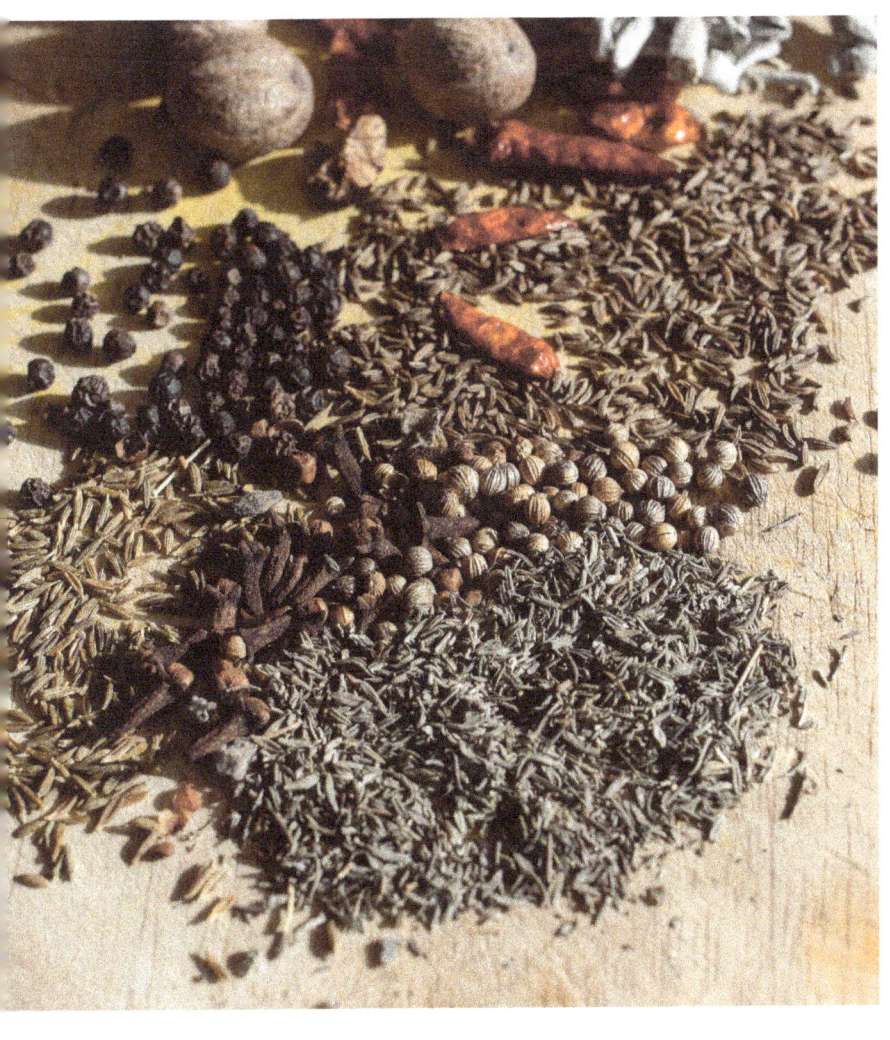

Freekeh

Freekeh is a carefully roasted or smoked green grain from young durum wheat and more expensive than bulgur. It originated in the Levantine area of the middle east and parts of North Africa.

Freekeh means that the wheat has been rubbed by both hands to remove the outer layer of skin after it has been roasted.

It has a delicious smokey, nutty flavour and is rich in proteins and minerals. It requires more cooking time than rice and bulgur but is less starchy than them. It needs to be slow cooked, taking over an hour.

During its processing, debris or small stones may be introduced to the freekeh, so it is important they are removed by hand prior to cooking. Afterwards, you place the freekeh in a large bowl of water in order to remove any floating debris, repeating this 2-3 times. Finally, remove the freekeh from the water by hand or sieve.

Just like pulses, freekeh tastes more delicious when eaten the day after cooking.

Good quality freekeh should have a green tint.

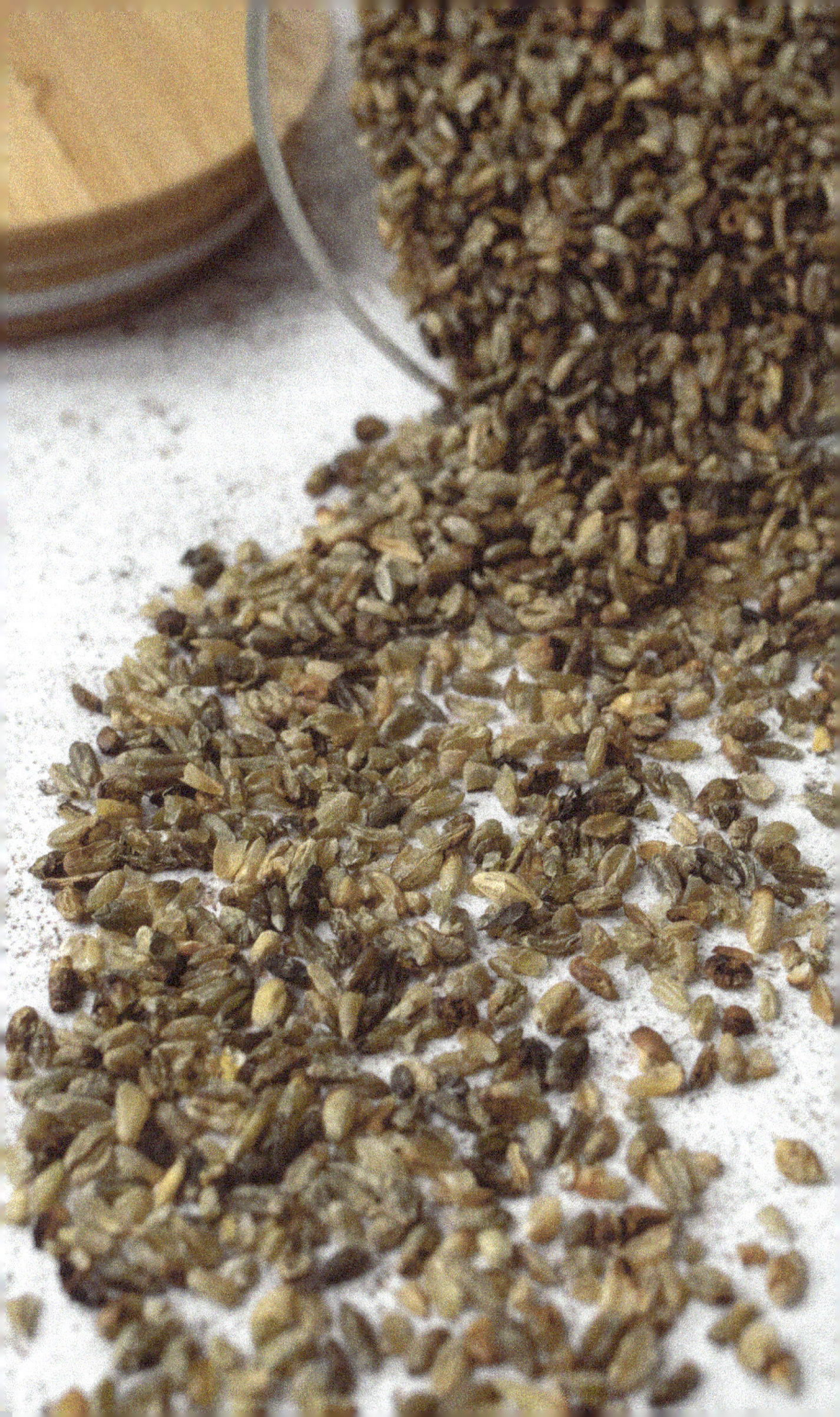

Freekeh with Mixed Nuts

3 cups freekeh

4 cups water

1 ½ tsp sea salt

2 tsp kabsa spices

2 finely chopped onions

2 chopped tomatoes

6 tbsp olive oil

¾ cup mixed nuts

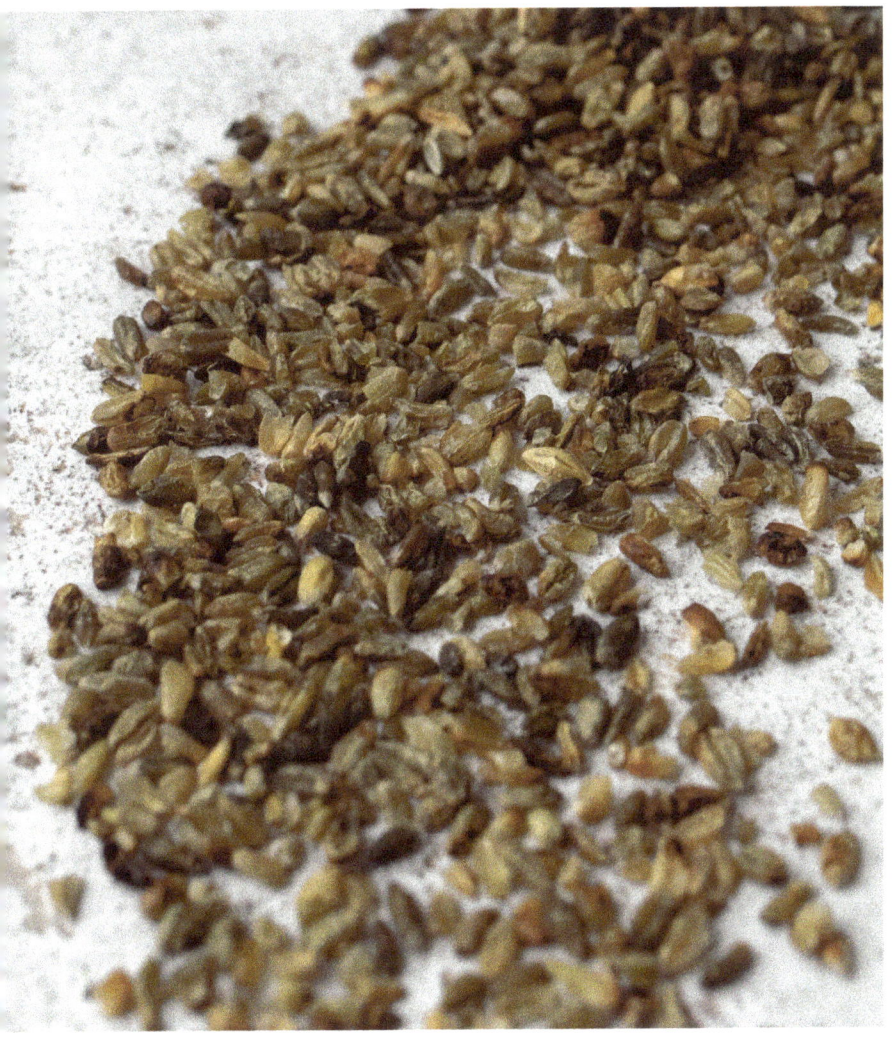

Preparation and Method

Prepare the freekeh as recommended on the 'Freekeh' page.

Heat 3 tbsp of olive oil in a saucepan. Add the onions and sauté until they become light golden. Then add the tomatoes, salt, kabsa spices and freekeh. Stir the mixture before adding the water and bring to the boil. Once boiling, turn the heat down and leave it to simmer for about 60-70 minutes.

Turn off the heat, add another 3 spoons of olive oil and the mixed nuts. Stir in and leave to rest for 10 minutes before serving. Serves 4

Tips: Serve with vegan tzatziki or with salad. For those with coeliac disease or gluten intolerance, replace freekeh with rice but you need to ensure that the ingredients are cooked before you add the rice because it takes less time to cook.

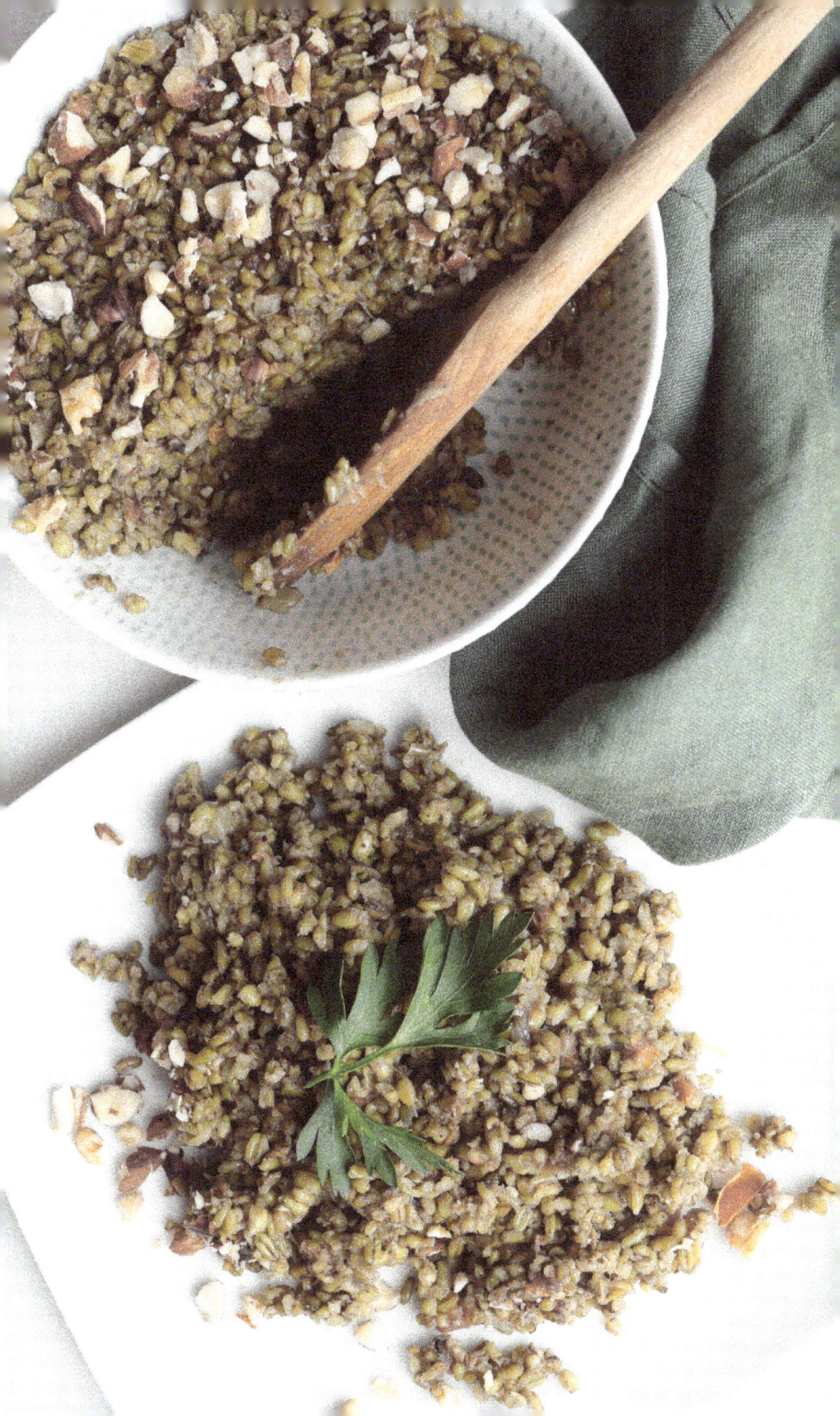

Vine Wraps Stuffed with Freekeh & Herbs

400g pickled vine leaves

2 ½ cups freekeh

1 cup grated vegan mozzarella cheese

4 small chopped tomatoes

2 cups finely chopped spring onions

2 cups chopped parsley

½ cup chopped fresh mint

½ cup chopped dill

¾ cup extra virgin olive oil

2 ¾ tsp sea salt

2 tbsp tomato purée

Juice of 1 lemon (optional)

2 cups boiled water

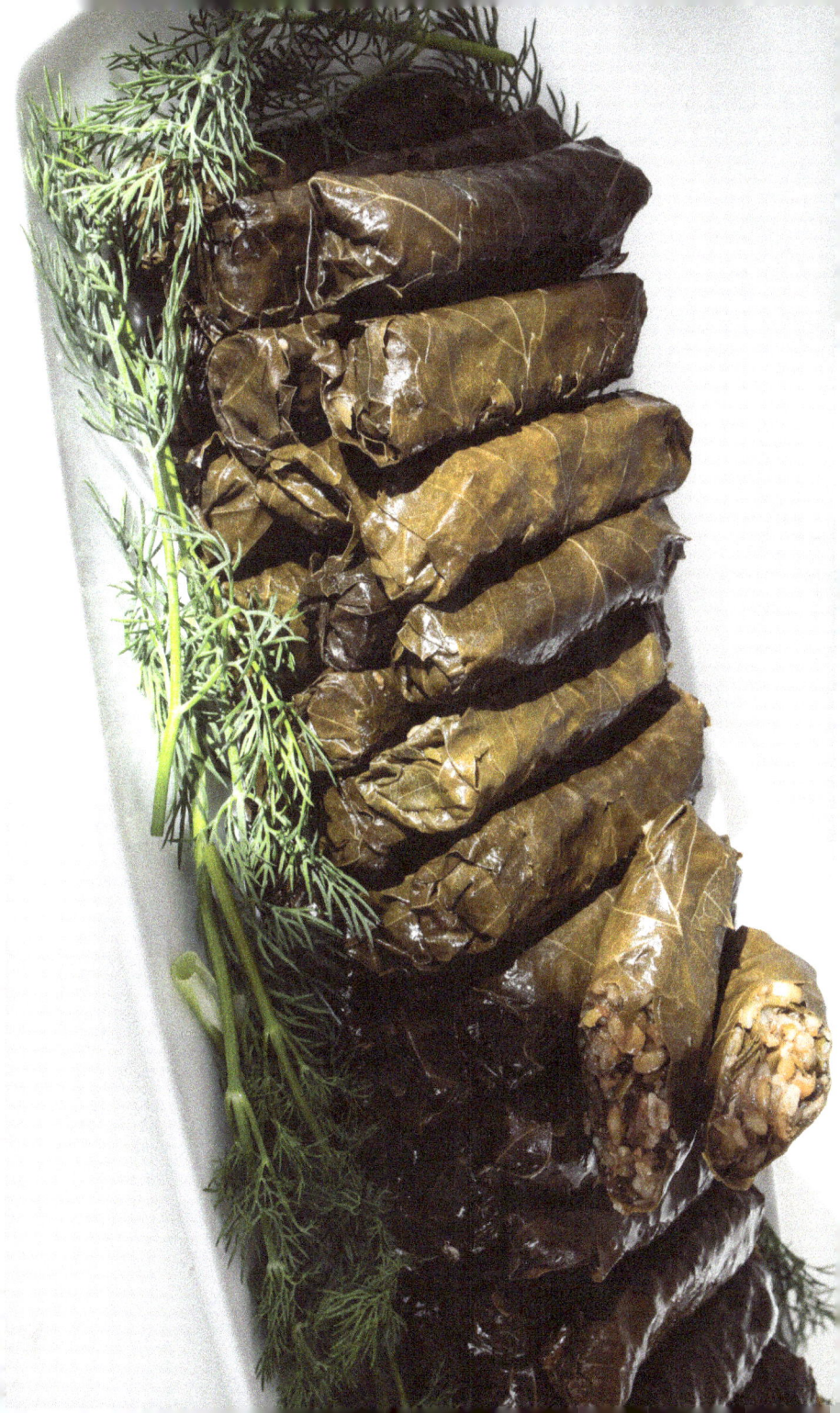

Preparation and Method

Wash the parsley, mint, spring onions and dill, then use a blender to chop them into small pieces. Prepare the freekeh as recommended on the page titled 'Freekeh' and mix in the parsley, mint, spring onions and dill by hand. Then add the cheese, salt, tomato purée and olive oil (leaving about 4 tbsp of olive oil aside). Cover and place the mixture in the fridge overnight.

The next day, the vine leaves need to be soaked in fresh water for about 2 hours before using to remove the salt that is used to preserve them.

Wrap each vine leaf around approx. 1 tbsp of the mixture. Start by opening the leaf out and placing the mixture in the center. Then you fold the left and right sides of the leaf inwards first, then roll from bottom to top, encompassing the contents securely in the vine leaf. This technique is similar to how you would fold a sandwich wrap. If you like, you can go online to find a video of how to achieve this technique.

Use a wide saucepan and place the wraps next to each other inside it. Add 2 cups of boiled water and cover the saucepan with the lid. Bring to boil and reduce to a low/medium heat to leave it to simmer for about 1 hour and 30 minutes.

Mix the lemon juice with 4 tbsp of olive oil and use as a dressing when finished.

Leave to rest for 5 minutes before you serve.

Serves 4-6

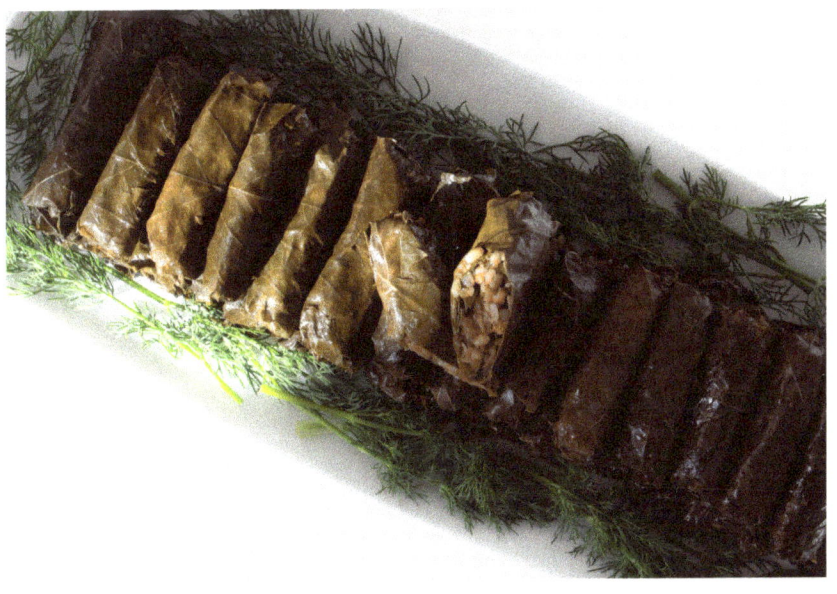

Stuffed Aubergines & Courgettes in Tomato Sauce

About 1kg baby aubergines & courgettes

¾ cup rice (brown or white)

1 cup finely chopped spring onion

1 cup chopped fresh parsley

3 finely chopped tomatoes

½ cup chopped fresh mint

½ tsp wild thyme

½ tsp black paper

1 tbsp tomato purée

3 crushed garlic cloves

1 tsp sea salt

¼ cup olive oil

1 cup vegan mozzarella grated cheese

Tomato Sauce Ingredients:

4 tomatoes

2 garlic cloves

½ tbsp tomato puree

2-3 tbsp olive oil

1 tsp cumin powder

1 cup water

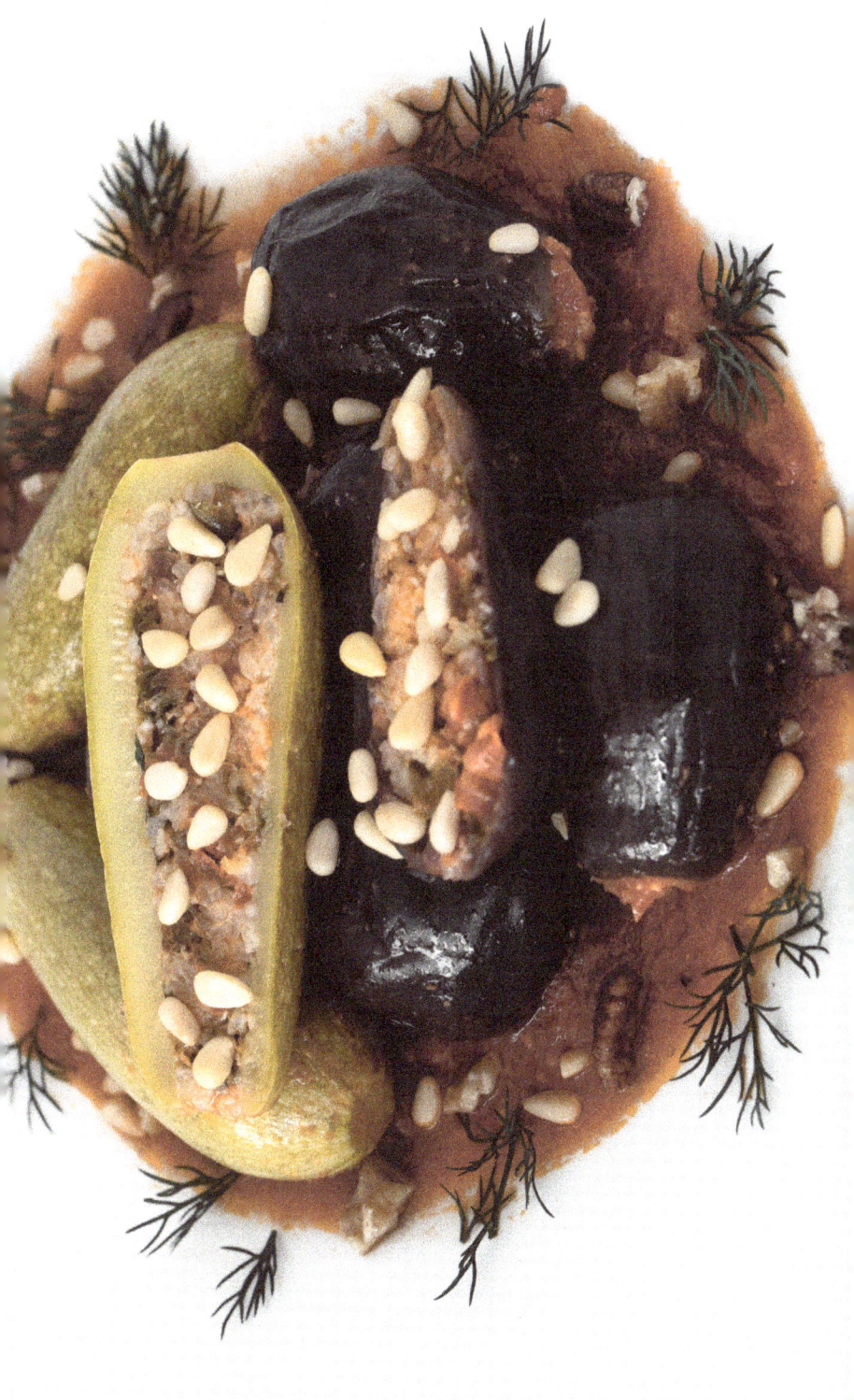

Preparation and Method

Add the herbs to the tomatoes, salt, cheese, tomato purée and olive oil and mix together with the rice and leave aside.

To make the tomato sauce, place all the ingredients under 'Tomato Sauce Ingredients' in a blender and blend until smooth.

Remove the insides of the courgettes and aubergines. Ensure at least 5mm thickness across the circumference of the courgettes to prevent it from splitting during cooking. Soak them in a solution of 3 tbsp of salt in 2 liters of water for about 30 minutes. After removing from the water, begin to stuff them with the mixture. Once done, place them in a large wide saucepan. Add the tomato sauce on top of the stuffed aubergines and courgettes, place the lid on top, bring to boil, then reduce to a medium heat and leave to simmer for about 45-60 minutes.

Serves 4

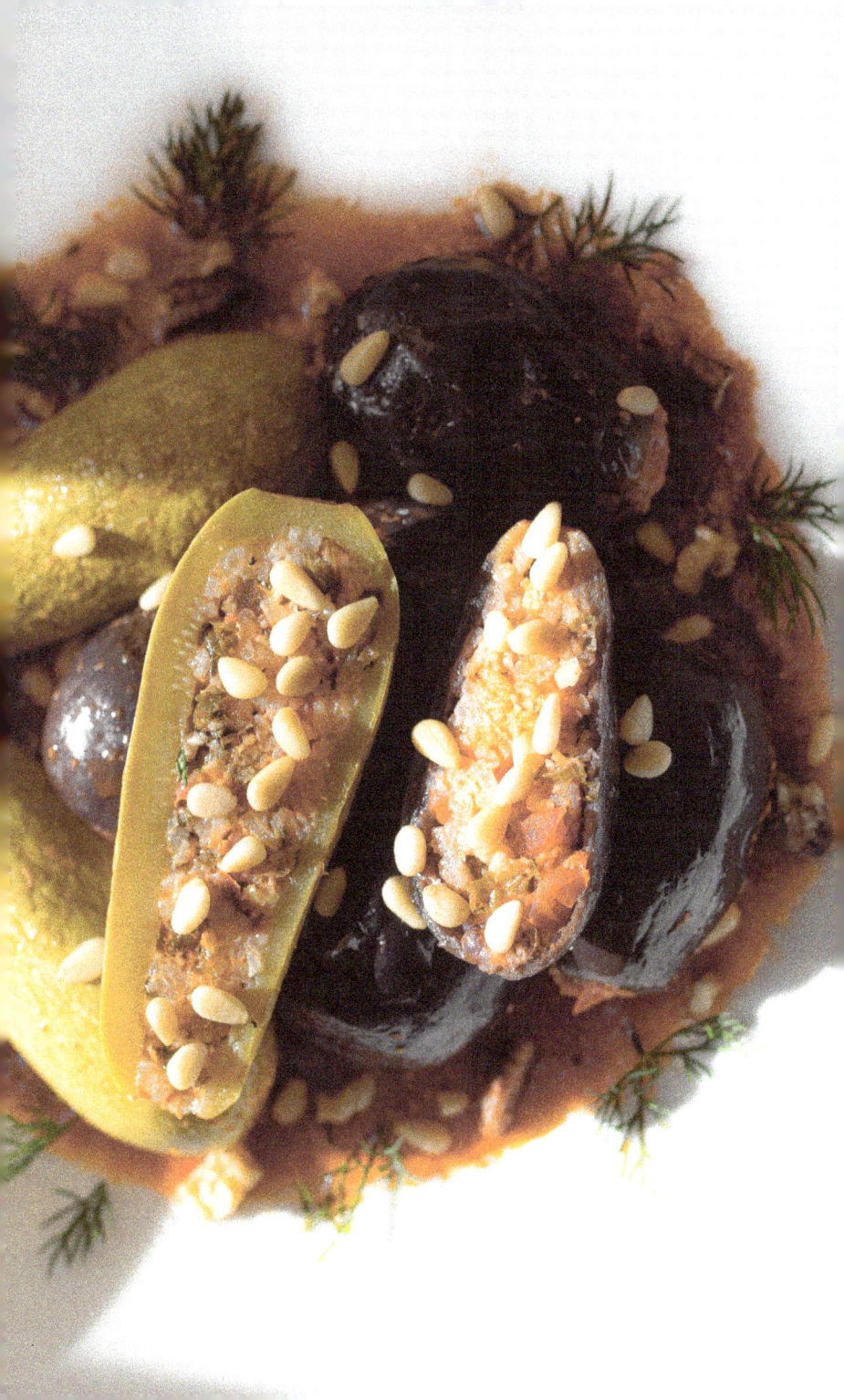

Cabbage Wraps

1 large sweetheart cabbage

1 cup short grain rice

1 ¼ tsp salt

1 cup chopped parsley

1/3 cup chopped dill

1/3 cup chopped mint

1 finely chopped small onion

4 crushed garlic cloves

2 tbsp tomato purée

¼ cup olive oil

1 lemon juice

1 cup grated vegan mozzarella cheese

½ cup boiled water

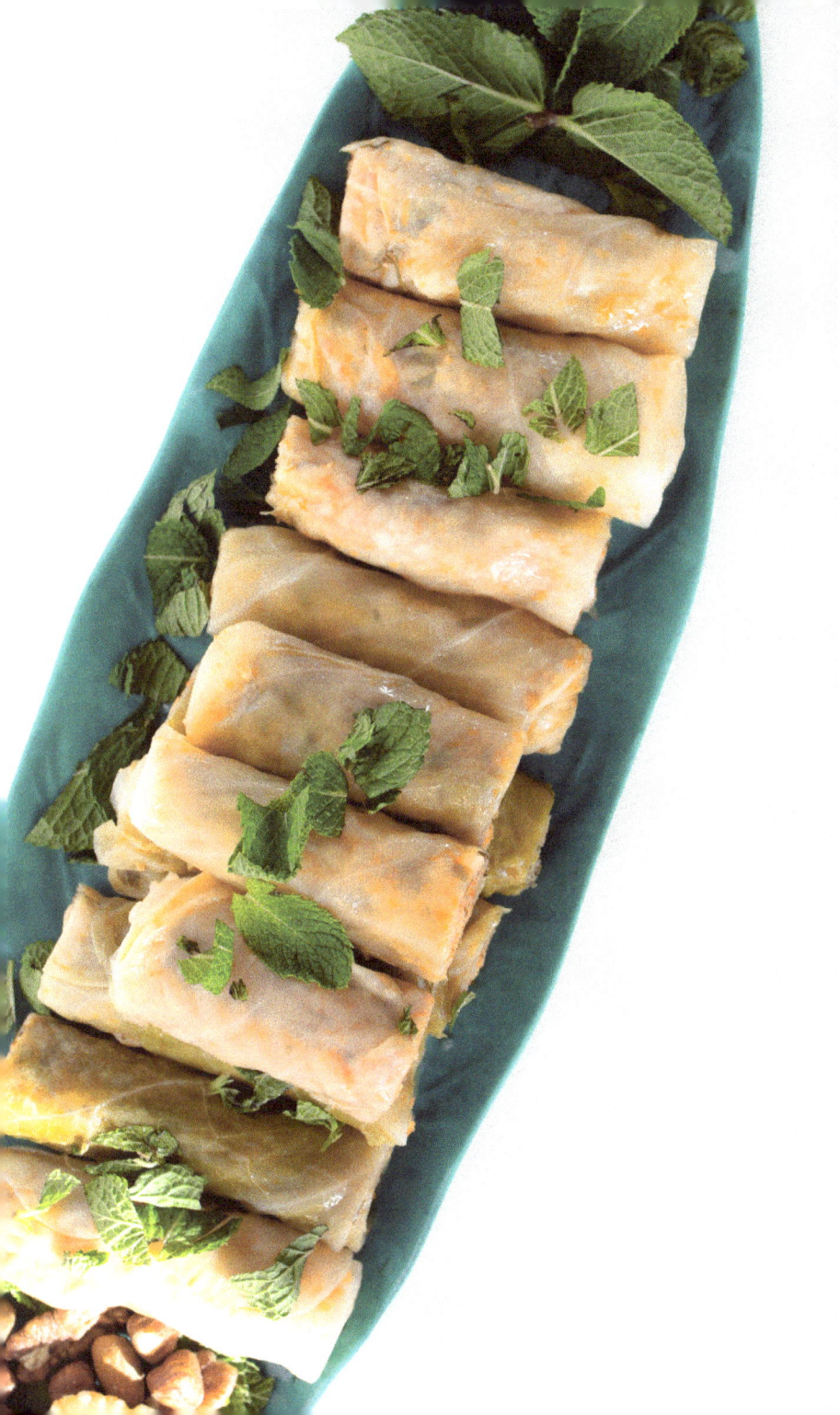

Preparation and Method

Carefully cut out the triangular core of the cabbage using a knife to allow you to peel apart the cabbage leaves without tearing. If you are unable to remove the individual leaves without tearing, then soak the whole cabbage in boiled water with 2 tbsp of salt for several minutes to allow you to remove them individually as they soften. Once all the leaves have been separated, place them back in the salty water for a couple of minutes until they wilt. This allows the leaves to be wrapped without tearing. Once done, remove from the water and stack ready to be wrapped. With large leaves cut into two sections, either side of the hard stem, discarding the hard stem.

Thoroughly mix the herbs, onion, garlic, tomato puree, oil, cheese, salt and rice in a bowl. Spread out the cabbage leaves on a chopping board and start filling with about 1 tbsp of mixture for each large leaf and less for smaller leaves. Wrap using the same technique explained in

'Vine Wraps Stuffed with Freekeh & Herbs' recipe and place tidily in a large saucepan. Once done, add ½ cup of boiled water, place the lid on, bring to boil, then reduce to medium/low heat and leave to simmer for 45-60 minutes. Before serving, dress with the lemon juice and some freshly chopped or dried mint.

Serves 3-4

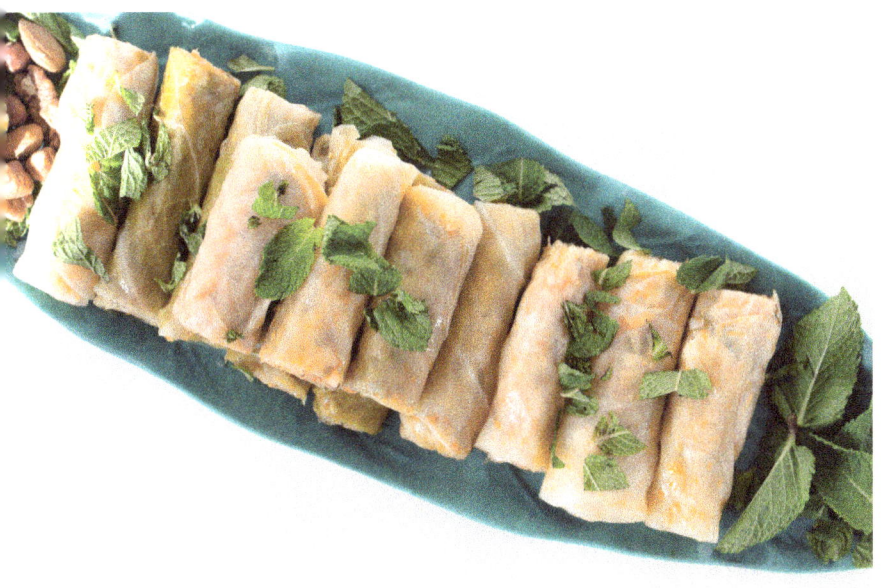

Barley

Barley is similar to other grains, rich in protein and some minerals such as iron and magnesium, as well as vitamin B6.

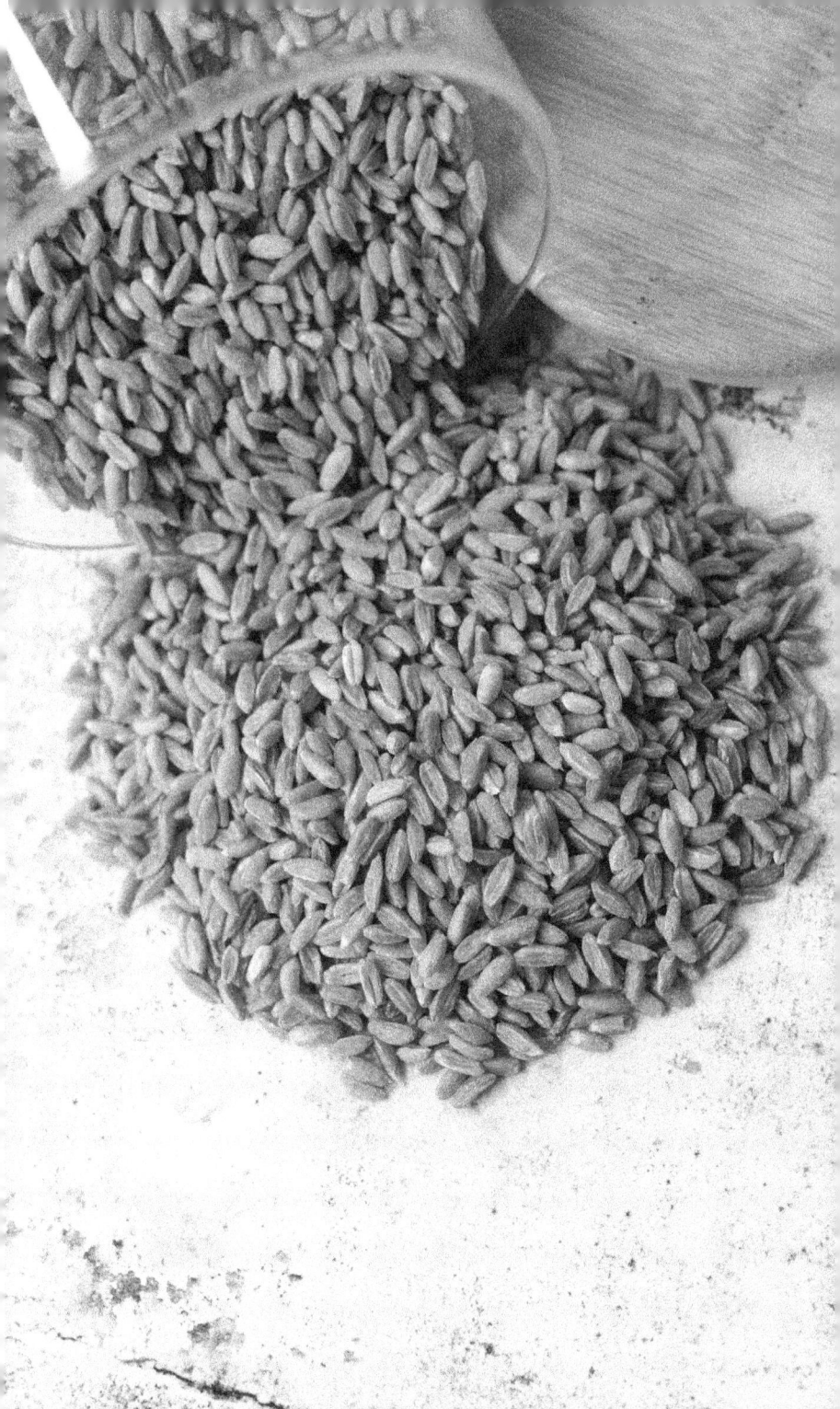

Baked Vegan Burgers

1 medium size boiled potato

1 cup dried peas soaked in water overnight

2 cups boiled barley

¼ cup olive oil

¼ cup coconut oil (melted)

1 small sized onion

3 garlic cloves

1 tbsp wild dry thyme

½ tsp sage powder

2 tbsp chopped fresh dill

2 tbsp tomato purée

2 tsp sea salt

2 tsp smoked paprika

½ tsp black pepper

¼ tsp red chili powder

1 tbsp cornflour

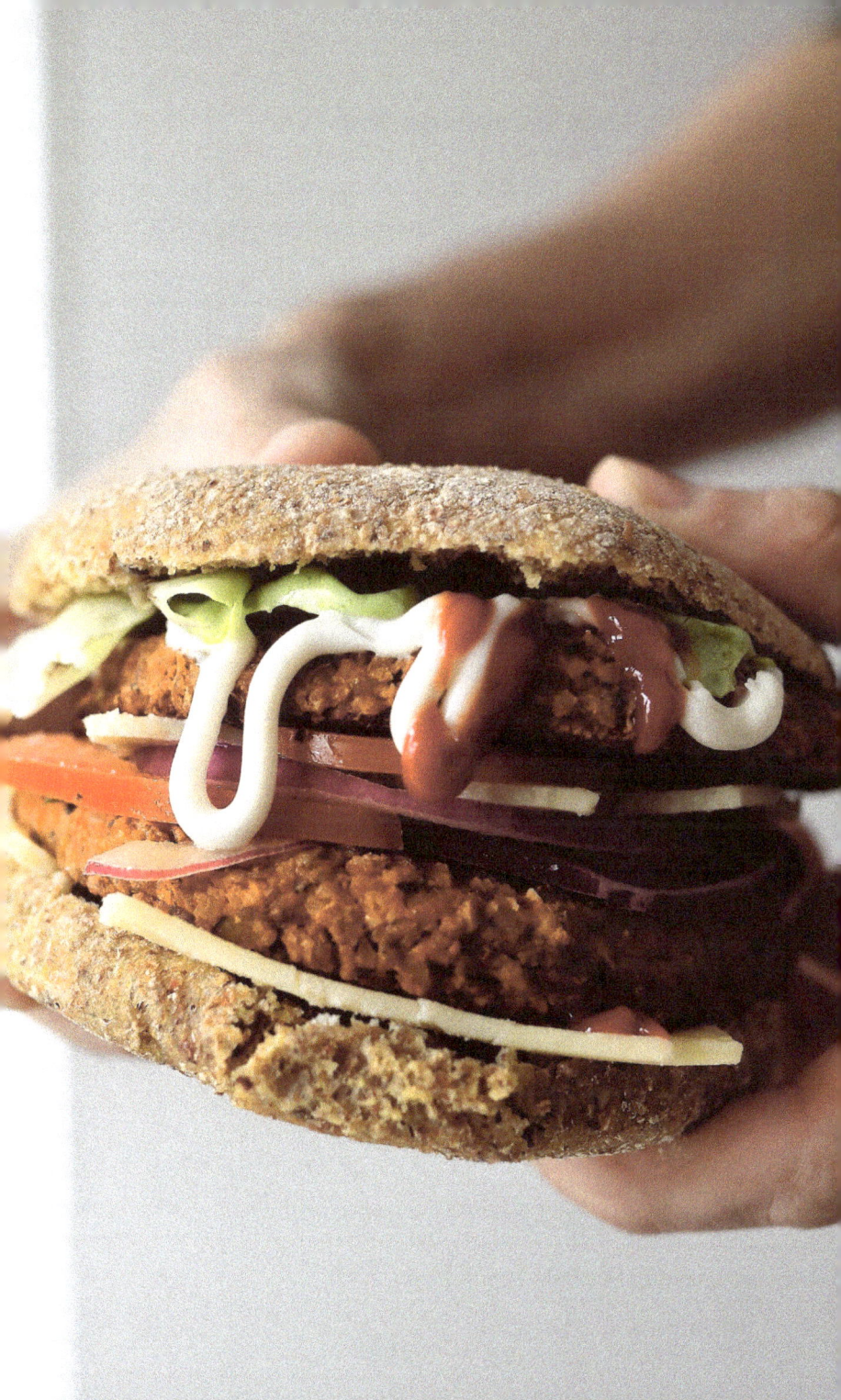

Preparation and Method

Boil the potato and mash it. Put the boiled barley and mashed potato into a large bowl and mix together. Drain and rinse the peas and place into a blender with the rest of the ingredients (excluding the barley, potato and coconut oil) and blend into a smooth paste. Add this paste to the barley and potato mixture. Then add the melted coconut oil and mix together by hand thoroughly before cooking. Brush an oven tray with coconut oil. Mould the mixture into burger patty's and place them on the tray. Brush the top of the burgers with coconut oil before cooking.

Preheat the oven to 180°C and place the tray in the middle of the oven. Cook for 20 minutes then flip them over, reduce the heat to 150°C and leave to cook for another 15 minutes.

Switch off the oven and leave them inside to rest for 10 minutes before you serve.

Delicious when served with hummus dip or salad.

Serves 4-5

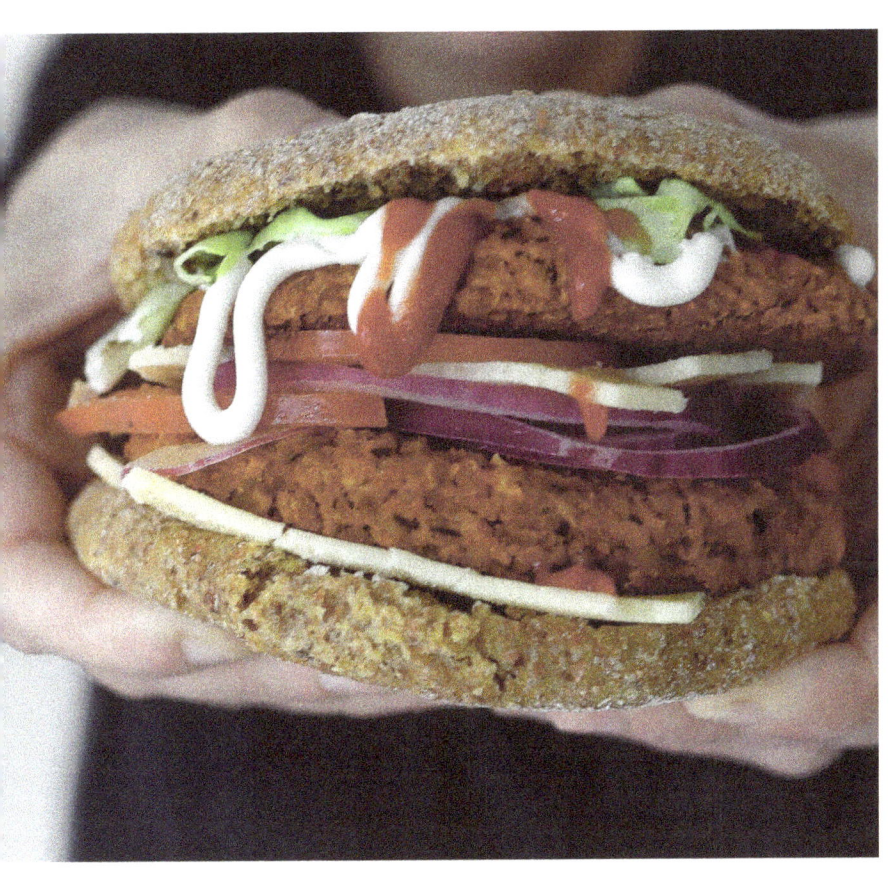

Barley with Lentil & Crunchy Peanut Butter

1 ½ cups boiled barley

1 ½ cups boiled lentils

3 medium tomatoes chopped into cubes

½ large cucumber cut into cubes

2 ½ tbsp crunchy peanut butter (with no added sugar)

2 crushed garlic cloves

3 tbsp olive oil

Juice of 1 squeezed lemon or lime

1 tsp sea salt

¼ tsp chili powder

1 tbsp cider vinegar

½ cup chopped mint

½ cup crispy onions (usually found near the spices section in supermarkets)

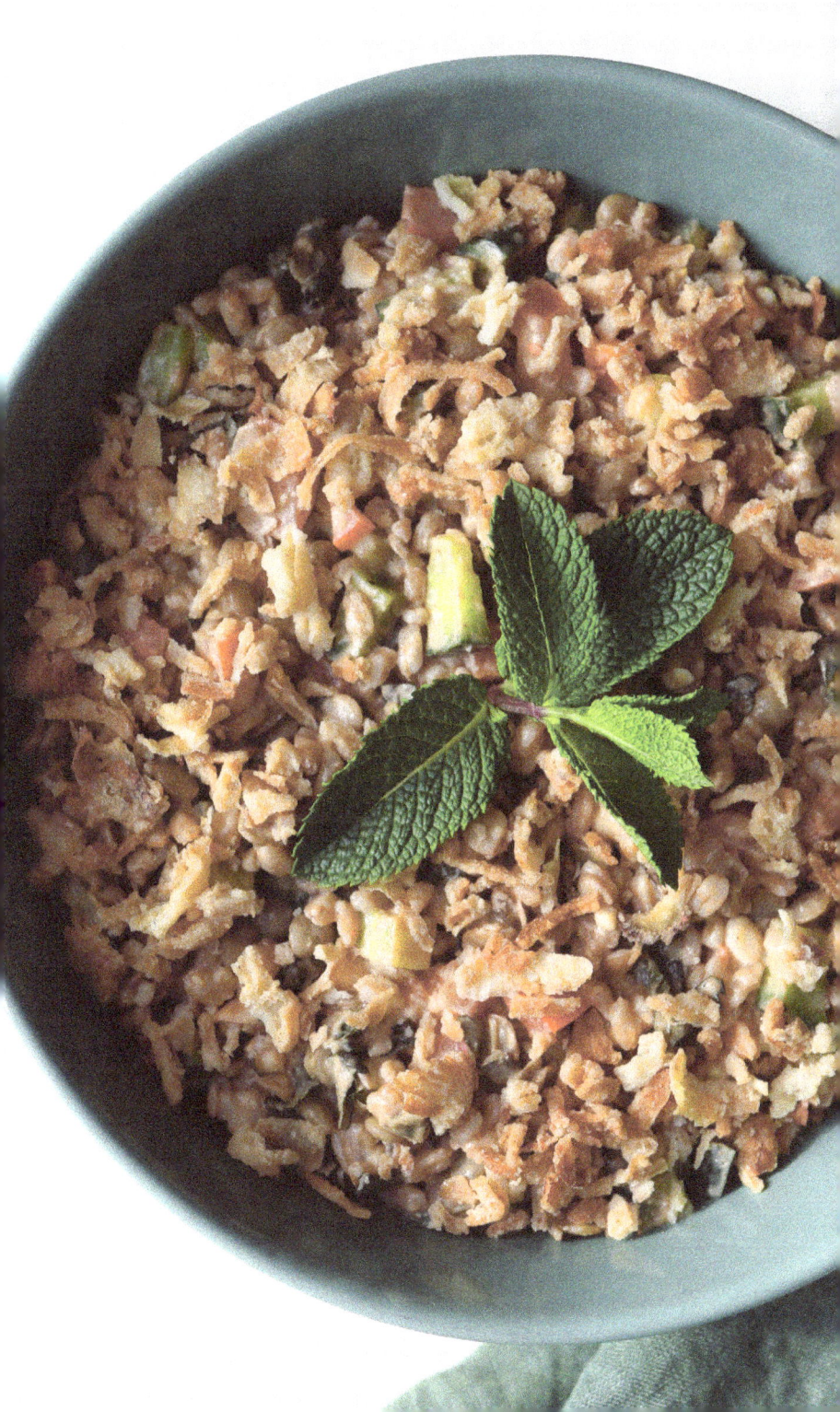

Preparation and Method

Put the peanut butter, lemon juice, garlic, vinegar, olive oil, salt, mint and chili powder together into a large bowl and mix thoroughly. Then add the cucumber and tomatoes. Finally, add the barley, lentils and crispy onions. Sprinkle some crispy onion on top.

Serves 3-4

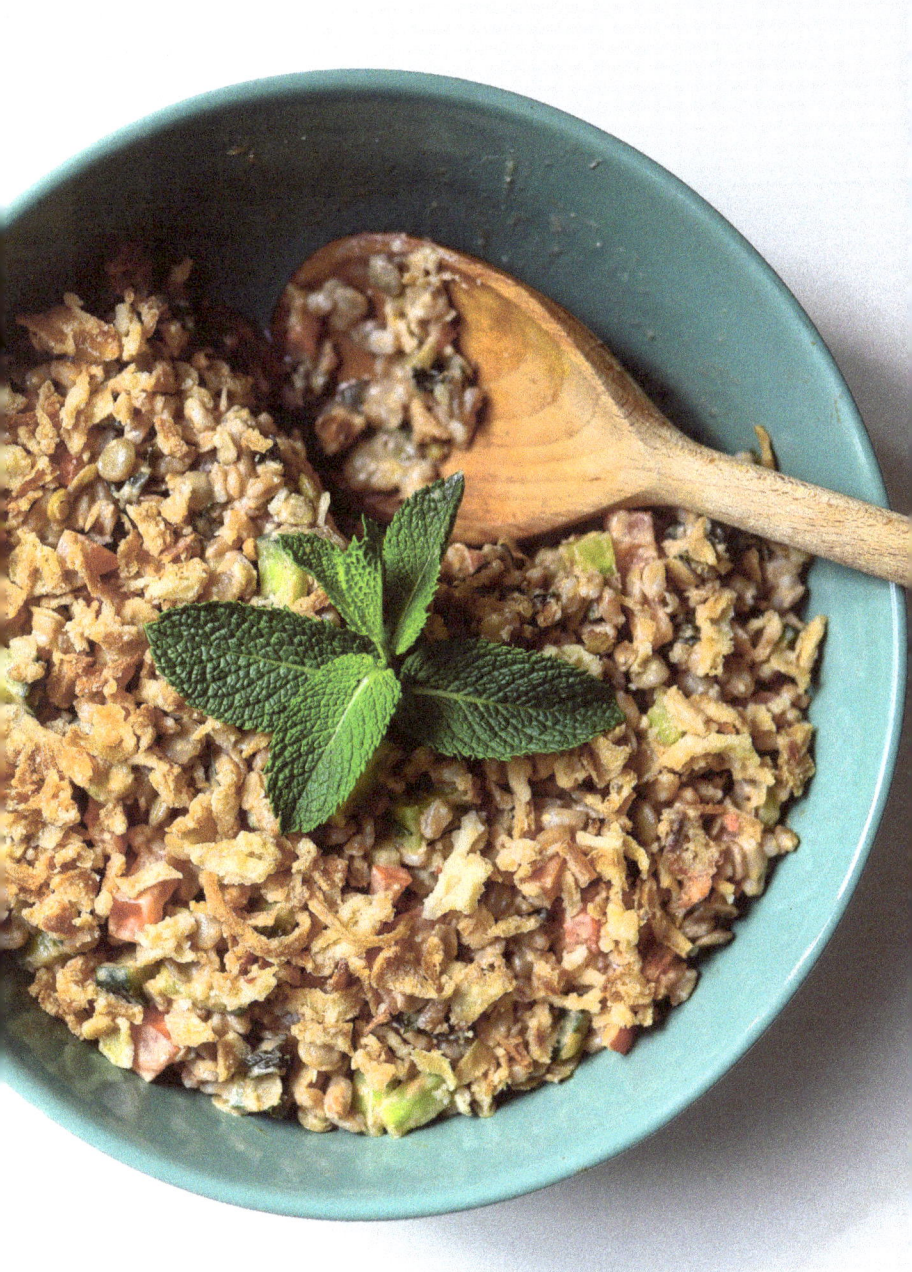

Soya Mince

Soya mince is processed from soya beans and is considered to have a good amount of protein and fibre.

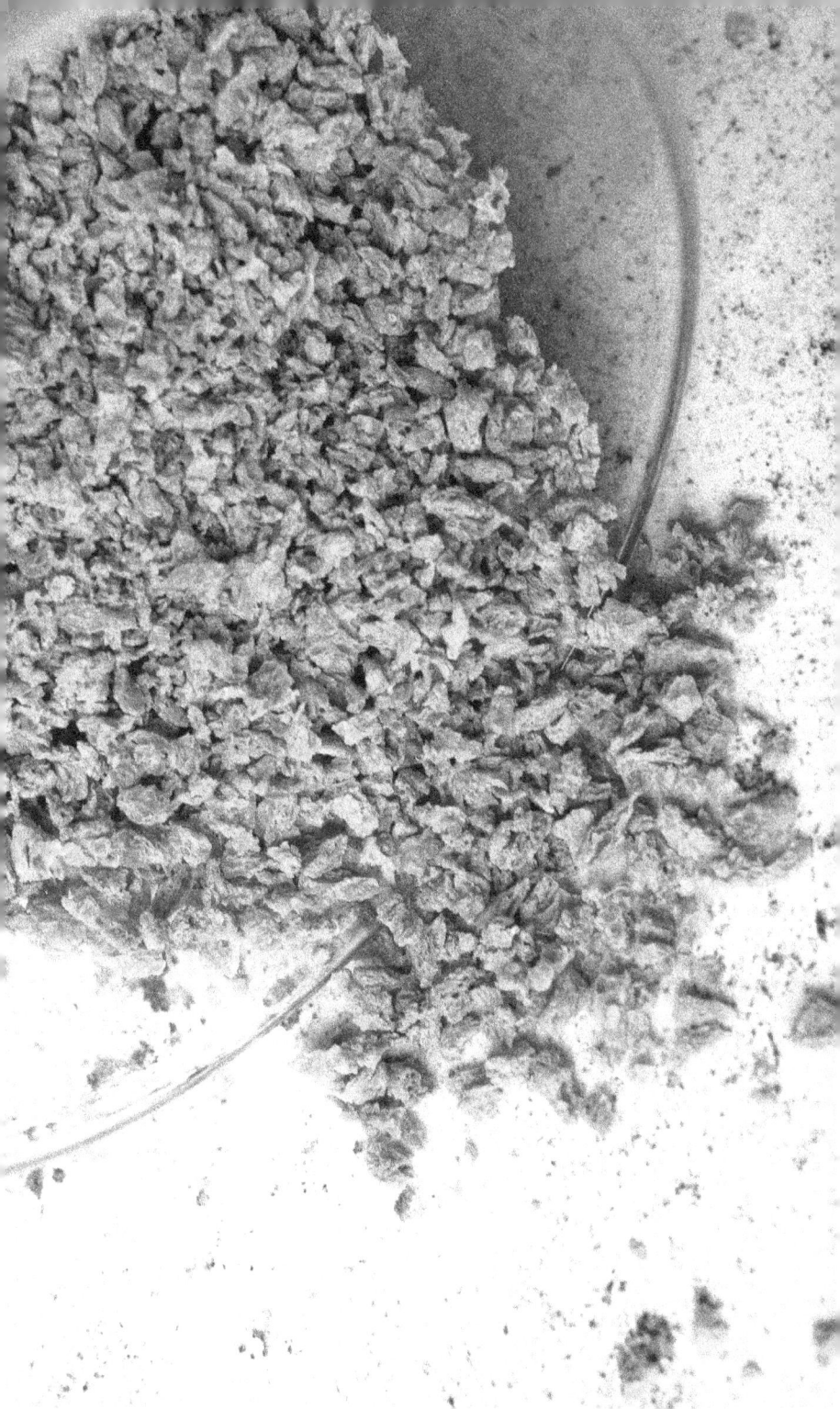

Grilled Vegan Kafta

3 cups boiled spelt barley (barley should not be over boiled or mushy)

1 ½ cups soya mince

100g minced mushroom

100g grated vegan mozzarella cheese

1 ¼ cups chopped green coriander

1 small finely chopped onion

3 crushed garlic cloves

2 tbsp tomato purée

1 tbsp kabsa spices

1 tbsp cornflour

1 tsp sea salt

1 tbsp coconut oil (melted)

3 tbsp olive oil

Wooden skewers (optional)

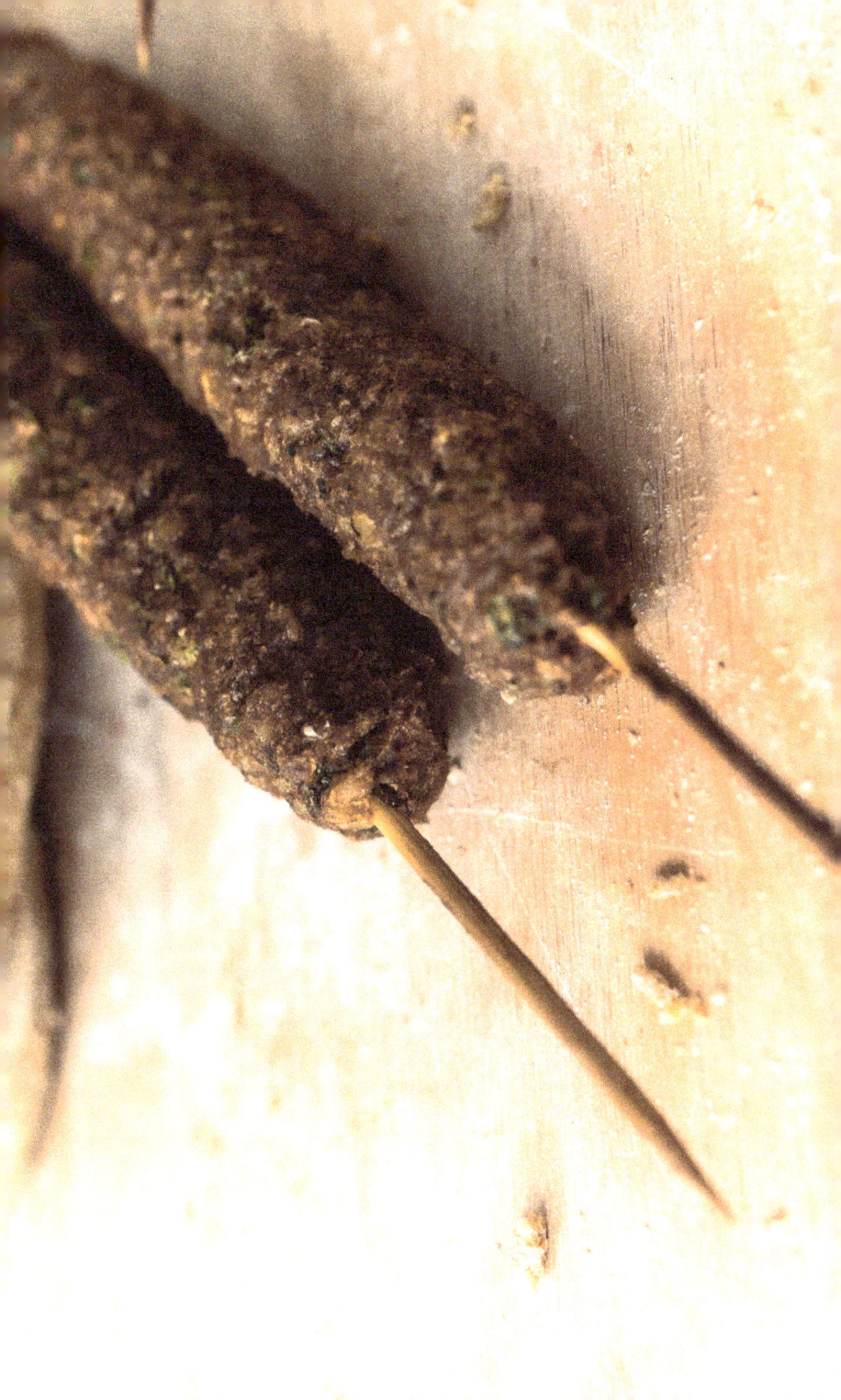

Preparation and Method

Put the barley in a blender and blend until the barley has broken down roughly into halves. Then empty into a large bowl. Add the other ingredients and mix them thoroughly together by hand until a dough-like consistency is formed. Cover the bowl and place in the fridge for at least one hour.

Prepare for grilling by separating a small amount of the mixture (the size of a large egg), roll it in your palm and wrap it fairly thinly around a wooden skewer as pictured.

When the skewers are ready, grill using the low heat setting for about 10 minutes on both sides. Leave to cool for 10 minutes before serving. Serves 4-5

Note: Mixture can be rolled into thin sausage-like structures without the use of skewers.

Tip: Delicious to be served with aubergine or hummus dip.

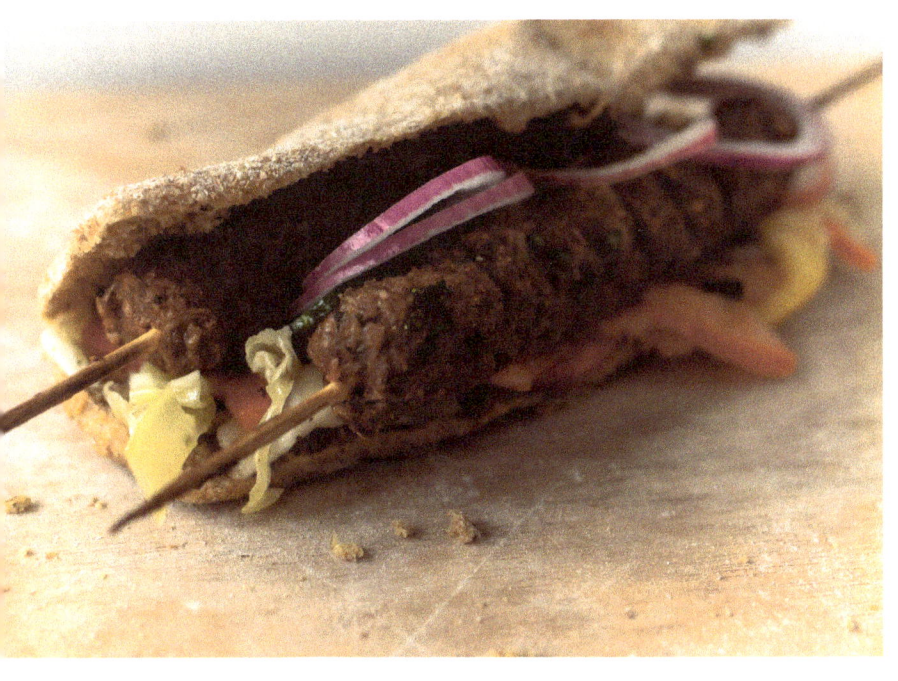

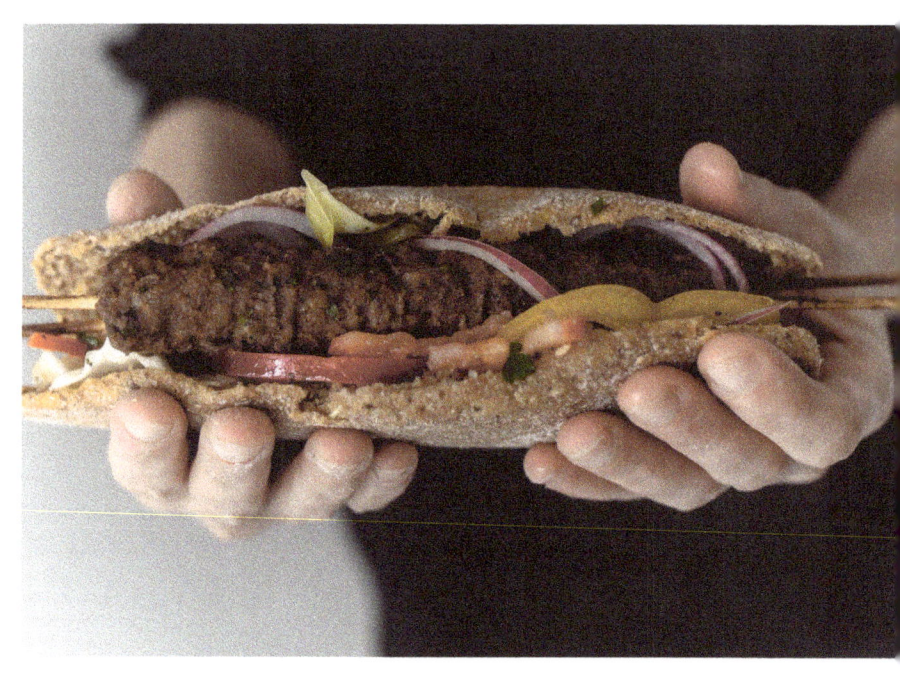

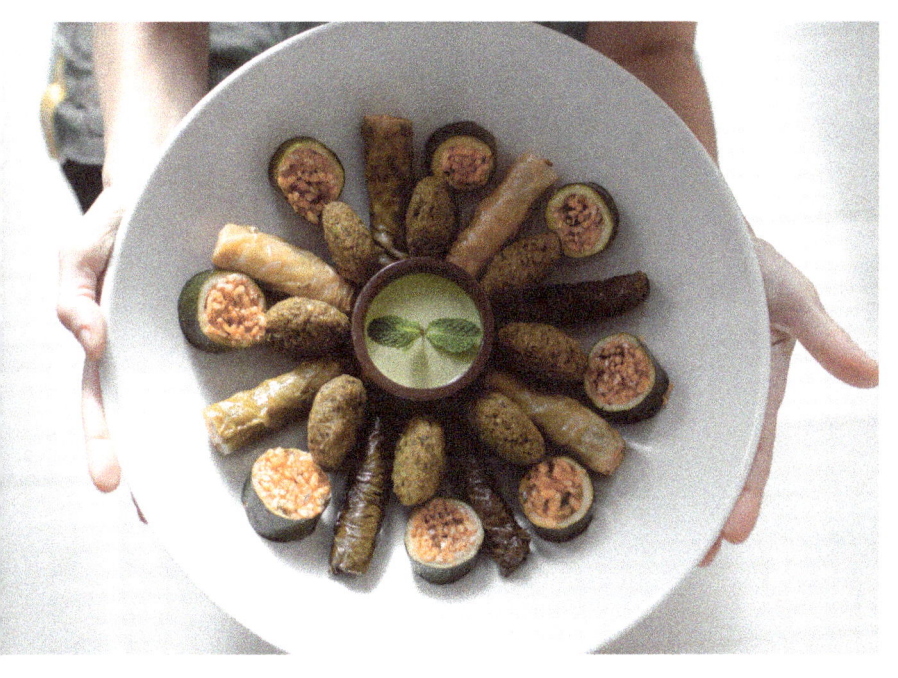

www.ingramcontent.com/pod-product-compliance
Lightning Source LLC
Chambersburg PA
CBHW040415100526
44588CB00022B/2839